LIVE AND LAUGH
WITH DEMENTIA

To the people I enjoy laughing with the most
— Tim, Mei and Aileen

Lee-Fay Low is a leading researcher in the field of dementia, and is passionate about ensuring that people with dementia live good and happy lives. Currently Associate Professor in Ageing and Health at the University of Sydney, Dr Low has researched programs on humour therapy, music, dance, intergenerational care, and reablement. Her interest in dementia began close to home, as her grandmother had vascular dementia.

LIVE AND LAUGH WITH DEMENTIA

The essential guide to maximizing quality of life

LEE-FAY LOW
BSC PSYCH (HONS) PHD

Empower

practical self-help tools by leading experts

'It is important to understand that dementia is as much a social issue as it is a medical one.

The essential part of understanding dementia is to recognise the importance of everyday relationships and empowering people with dementia to live well though good support in the community. It also means having dementia-friendly organisations to access services such as banking, retail and Centrelink. Humour too, is a critical part of the journey; learning to laugh with people with dementia is important in coming to terms with the diagnosis.

This insightful book focuses on what is important in the everyday life of the person with dementia and the family carer and explores the practical things we can all do to make our communities more dementia friendly.'

Glenn Rees AM, Chair, Alzheimer's Disease International

'A book full of wonderful gifts of knowledge.'

Nurses Net

'... an amazing inspiring manual of making life with dementia as positive as possible ... She writes with enthusiasm and insight. It's a book full of wonderful gifts of knowledge.'

Nursing Times

'... I was amazed and delighted by the number and profundity of the insights it contains. It is packed with very good advice about communication, activities, and relationships, and I cannot imagine any carer not benefiting from it hugely.'

Australian Journal of Dementia

'*Live and Laugh with Dementia* is not only easy to read but will speak to the heart of occupational therapists as Lee-Fay commences by emphasising the importance of meaningful activities for persons with dementia. This is a very informative book for those who are new to the field of dementia care; or could serve as encouragement to experts and a means to support their approach to practice if they are keen to promote client-directed care.

This is the first book since the publication of Perrin, May, Anderson's 2008 publication, *Wellbeing in Dementia: An occupational approach for therapists and carers*, that I feel reflects the ethos of meaningful engagement where activity involvement is key. I hope that occupational therapists will be challenged and inspired by Lee-Fay to elaborate on the importance of supporting persons with dementia as occupational beings to experience quality of life.'

Sanet du Toit PhD, lecturer, Occupational Therapy Division,
University of Sydney

'... a how-to-guide to strengthen and maintain the mental and relationship muscles of the person with dementia ... a mix of science, experience, case studies, suggested activities and room for notes.'

Agendas: Aged and Community Services Australia Magazine

'A great resource ... Broken into logical sequences with easy to read tables of activities and clear concise language ...'

Fifty Plus News

First published 2014. This edition published 2018.

Exisle Publishing Pty Ltd
PO Box 864, Chatswood, NSW 2057, Australia
226 High Street, Dunedin, 9016, New Zealand
www.exislepublishing.com

A CiP record for this book is available from the
National Library of Australia.

ISBN 978-1-925335-72-9

Designed by Tracey Gibbs
Cover illustrations adapted from images
   courtesy of VectorStock
Typeset in MillerText
Printed in China

This book uses paper sourced under ISO 14001
guidelines from well-managed forests and other
controlled sources.

10 9 8 7 6 5 4 3 2 1

Disclaimer

This book is a general guide only and should never be a substitute for the skill, knowledge and experience of a qualified medical professional dealing with the facts, circumstances and symptoms of a particular case. The nutritional, medical and health information presented in this book is based on the research, training and professional experience of the author, and is true and complete to the best of their knowledge. However, this book is intended only as an informative guide; it is not intended to replace or countermand the advice given by the reader's personal physician. Because each person and situation is unique, the author and the publisher urge the reader to check with a qualified health care professional before using any procedure where there is a question as to its appropriateness. Your health care practitioner should be consulted before beginning any new treatment program, including diet, lifestyle and/or physical activity. The author, publisher and their distributors are not responsible for any adverse effects or consequences resulting from the use of the information in this book. It is the responsibility of the reader to consult a physician or other qualified healthcare professional regarding their personal care. This book contains references to products and procedures that may not be available everywhere. The intent of the information provided is to be helpful; however, there is no guarantee of results associated with the information provided. Use of drug brand names is for educational purposes only and does not imply endorsement.

CONTENTS

INTRODUCTION:
USE IT OR LOSE IT

We exercise our body's muscles to keep them strong, flexible and working well. Similarly, we need to keep exercising our mental muscles (our brain) to keep them strong, flexible and working well. We also need to keep exercising our relationship muscles (our social networks and friendships) to keep them strong, flexible and working well. This is what *Live and Laugh with Dementia* is all about — strengthening and maintaining the mental and relationship muscles of the person with dementia for whom you care. The engaging philosophy and the suggested activities in this book will, I hope, help you provide positive experiences for that person.

This book is based on my experiences working with people with dementia and their carers, and on scientific research. I am an expert on dementia in general, but the best expert on the person with dementia you are looking after is you, their carer. Therefore, this is not a manual for you to follow exactly to guarantee activities that will engage a person with dementia. I need you to add two key ingredients to the information in this book: *your knowledge about the person with dementia* and *your creativity in selecting and modifying activities.* The information you have about the person's individual abilities and interests will help you choose the activities that they will be interested in and enjoy, and will help you modify them so that they can participate in them. Using ideas and inspiration from the book, you will tailor activities for the person and how you present them in order to successfully engage the person with dementia.

I've learnt from training professional carers that reflecting on personal experiences, writing down information about the person with dementia, and planning potential activities helps successfully create and implement activities. The worksheets included in this book should help you process and apply the information you've read.

I hope that in bringing pleasure to the person with dementia through activities, you will also derive happiness and satisfaction, and that through sharing smiles and activities your relationship will continue to grow.

CASE STUDIES

The stories that I share with you in this book are based on real people, though their names and details have been changed. We will meet Joy, who sings enthusiastically even though she can't remember doing so afterwards. Then there's Brian, who smiles and laughs even though he can't express himself with words very well. Ruth gives her visitor a warm welcoming cuddle even though she can't describe exactly who she is or how she knows her visitor. And Antonio talks animatedly even though he doesn't always make sense to others. Through the case studies we will see the ideas presented in this book put into practice.

WHY ENGAGE PEOPLE LIVING WITH DEMENTIA THROUGH MEANINGFUL ACTIVITIES?

Research has shown that there are a number of good reasons to do this:

- Activities provide mental and physical stimulation, which can slow decline or improve mental function.
- Activities are pleasurable.
- Activities are a way to develop or maintain a relationship.
- Activities help stave off boredom.
- Activities distract from behaviours that are difficult for carers.
- Activities help the person with dementia maintain their self-identity.

Let's look at each of these points in more detail.

Activities provide mental and physical stimulation, which can slow decline or improve mental function

Scientists used to think that the number of brain cells, or neurons, we had at birth was the maximum number we could have, and as brain cells died the number decreased through life. We now know that we grow new neurons throughout life, and that these new brain cells, and the important connections between the cells (known as neural pathways), grow in response to experiences in life such as learning new things or living in a mentally stimulating environment.

Mental activity, or mental exercise, encourages growth of new cells and strengthens connections between cells in the brain. There is good research evidence that cognitive stimulation therapy (discussed in detail in Chapter 5) improves or maintains cognition at a level similar to that achieved with the currently available drugs for Alzheimer's disease. This suggests that undertaking a variety of activities that use different mental abilities is good for people with dementia.

Physical activity, or physical exercise, builds and strengthens muscles of the body. It also seems to improve brain functioning, with a growing body of evidence suggesting that physical activity can improve memory and slow down cognitive decline in people with dementia. It seems that physical exercise can also stimulate neuronal growth, improving the neural efficiency of the brain, meaning that after exercise the brain uses less energy to do the same task. We think that physical exercise improves how well the brain runs. Physical activity may also have indirect effects on the brain by improving physical health. Physical exercise decreases blood pressure, cholesterol and depression, and reduces the effects of diabetes. All these health conditions are known to impact brain health.

Activities are pleasurable

Pleasure is the in-the-moment feeling of happiness in response to an external event, such as laughing with a child or relishing a piece of chocolate. Experiencing emotions is a fundamental part of being human, and happiness is one of the most basic emotions. It is the second emotion that babies express clearly through a smile at about six weeks of age, the first being distress or discomfort expressed through crying.

Experiencing pleasure is its own reward, but it is sometimes given a low priority. When we are busy caring for another person's medical and physical needs, it sometimes seems less important to spend time thinking about and organizing something that is enjoyable and fun. Remember that we also should try to look after their emotional needs, including needs for love, belonging and pleasure.

Most of us do some activities that bring us pleasure and enjoyment. Often, we do these activities in our spare time for fun or recreation and think of them as sport or a hobby or a pastime; some lucky people find work enjoyable too. People living with dementia have fewer opportunities to participate in activities that they find pleasurable. They have fewer opportunities to experience enjoyment, pleasure, joy, a sense of achievement, gratification, amusement, satisfaction, play or fun. The symptoms of dementia mean that they are unable to complete many of the pleasurable activities they previously enjoyed, and they also lose their ability to initiate pleasurable activities.

Certain chemicals are released in the brain when a person experiences the states of pleasure, happiness or contentment. These neurochemicals (endorphins, oxytocins, dopamine, serotonin) stay at higher levels in the brain even after the event that triggered the emotion has passed. That's why we continue to feel happy, even if less intensely so, after leaving a great party, a funny movie or spending time with a loved one. A build-up of many moments of pleasure, happiness and contentment accumulate to more general feelings of satisfaction with life, which is the state of happiness. There are many benefits of being happy. Happy people have better mental health, live longer, have better immune systems and tolerate pain better. Research suggests that in order to flourish psychologically we need to experience three positive emotions for every one negative emotion. This 'three positive to one negative' ratio seems also to apply to people with dementia.

I have been told on a few occasions that there is no point

doing activities with people with dementia since they don't remember them. I disagree. This is like saying there is no point behaving lovingly to babies until the age of three because we don't remember events before the age of three. Each experience in our lives changes us in some small way each time. An accumulation of positive life experiences tends to give a person a more positive outlook. This is partly because we remember those experiences, and also because our patterns of behaviour and structures in our brain are cumulatively changed by those experiences. A person with dementia often will not remember the details of an activity, or the activity at all, but this does not mean that the activity does not make a difference to his or her life.

Activities are a way to develop or maintain a relationship

A relationship is a connection, association or involvement between persons. Friendship is a type of relationship in which two people voluntarily spend mutually enjoyable time together.

If you are a family member or friend of the person with dementia for whom you are caring, then the nature of your past relationship will affect how you interact now. You will probably have expectations of how your loved one should behave as your husband, wife, parent or friend, and he or she may have expectations of how you should behave. However, your role as carer, and the person's disease and symptoms, mean that by necessity the nature of your relationship has changed. You most probably feel a sense of loss and sadness at this change in your relationship. Doing activities together is a way to maintain your relationship, and some activities may even help it feel more normal.

We often maintain relationships and friendships through

conversation. When we 'catch up' with old friends we usually talk about news of what has happened since our last meeting, and sometimes reminisce about experiences we have shared together. People with dementia find it increasingly difficult to have these types of catching-up conversations. Their poor memories mean that they can't remember the answers to commonly asked questions, or report news. They may become upset or confused when trying to remember. The other mental challenges that dementia brings mean that people with dementia also have trouble finding the right words, can lose track of what they were saying, and as dementia progresses may have trouble forming sentences or talking at all. However, people with dementia report that friendships are important to them, and they conceptualize friendships in the same way other adults do.

Activities are a way we can maintain relationships. Sharing experiences brings people closer emotionally, particularly when strongly emotional experiences are shared. This is why soldiers often develop deep bonds. Your past and current relationship may affect the choice of activities you do with the person with dementia, and how you introduce the activities. For instance, if your loved one was bossy and still expects to make decisions, then choose an activity where she can demonstrate her expertise or has a lot of choice and control, rather than an activity where she needs to rely on your help a lot.

If you are a new person involved in the person with dementia's life, either as a friend, volunteer or paid carer, you need to get to know them. However, our usual strategies for getting to know someone by asking questions about them often do not work with a person with dementia because of their poor memory. You can get to know a person with dementia and form a relationship with them by doing activities together. As you do activities, you will see patterns of behaviour that show their personality and reveal what they like and dislike. You will both develop patterns of interacting. You can build a connection with the person with dementia without knowing many facts about them, in the same way that we sometimes connect with someone through shared activities such as a class or sport but don't know many facts about the rest of their lives.

Activities help stave off boredom

People with dementia often spend a lot of their time sitting around doing nothing. In nursing homes, the residents can spend up to 85 per cent of their time doing nothing. They report feeling bored, and they look and act disengaged from the world.

This boredom has consequences for the behaviour of people with dementia. We think that some of the agitated behaviours of persons with dementia such as pacing, wandering, calling out and screaming, repetitive talking or behaviour, restlessness and irritability arise because they are bored and have an unmet need for stimulation or company. Similarly, low mood and depression may also arise due to these unmet needs. Research shows that when people with dementia are engaged with meaningful activities they show reduced levels of agitated behaviours and better mood. You can think of activities as a preventative measure against these behaviours.

Activities distract from behaviours that are difficult for carers

People with dementia sometimes behave in ways that their carers find difficult to cope with. They can become physically or verbally aggressive. This may be because they have become upset or anxious because of a real event (such as a visit from someone they dislike), because they don't want to cooperate with something their carer asks them to do (such as having a shower), because of a false belief (such as thinking someone is stealing from them) or because of damage to brain structures caused by the disease.

Sometimes an activity can distract the person with dementia from the thing that upsets them and reduce their level of emotional distress and corresponding aggression. For example, going for a walk can take the person away from the distressing visitor, singing a happy song can change the mood in the bathroom and increase cooperation, and doing an activity that requires concentration such as sorting cards or doing some cooking together may stop the person with dementia ruminating about the thief.

Activities help the person with dementia maintain their self-identity

People with dementia have to live in the moment. The short-term and long-term memory loss that comes with dementia means that their lives are based on snapshots of 'now' rather than also being informed by past memories and future plans. People with dementia rely on the things they can see around them, and the way that they are treated by people around them, to tell them who they are in the world, and how things are. They are constantly interpreting the world around them to give meaning to their own situation. If people around them treat them with respect and happiness, they are more likely to feel like a respected and happy person. If they are ignored or criticized or disrespected, they will feel less valued or might get defensive.

Similarly, if people with dementia find themselves participating in an activity that is pleasurable and meaningful to them, then they will see themselves as being engaged with and able to impact their world.

1

HOW DEMENTIA AFFECTS THE WAY WE THINK

Dementia is the umbrella term for a group of conditions in which the brain deteriorates (see 'What the science tells us' on p. 27 if you are interested in the scientific details). In order to plan activities that a person with dementia can do, and help them participate as fully as possible in these activities, we need to understand the types of difficulties with thinking that people with dementia have and then create strategies to compensate for these difficulties.

Here are some of the abilities and characteristics handled by our brain:

- memory
- attention
- initiation
- decision making, problem solving and planning
- speech and comprehension
- perception — sight, sound, smell, touch
- our personality
- controlling our feelings
- controlling our movements.

Different areas of the brain are responsible for each ability listed, and all the abilities are affected by dementia.

DIFFICULTIES WITH MEMORY

There are two main types of memory: short-term and long-term. Short-term memory is information that we hold in our brain temporarily so that we can use the information fairly quickly. Examples include the name of a person we have just met at a party, or a telephone number that we want to dial. Most information that we store in our short-term memory we do not keep permanently, as our short-term memory store has a limited size. We can think of short-term memory as a holding room that can only store a maximum of between five and nine items of information. This maximum storage ability is sometimes referred to as 'seven plus or minus two'. We forget information when it is no longer useful to us, or when it is replaced by new items in our short-term store room.

Information is more permanently stored when it is transferred from our short-term memory to our long-term memory. We can consciously or unconsciously choose for this transfer to happen. An experience, piece of information or skill is more likely to be stored in our long-term memory if we have attended to it well, or practised or rehearsed it, if it is meaningful to us, and if it is associated with strong emotions (either good or bad).

People with dementia usually experience difficulties with their short-term memory first. They do not seem to be able to keep new information in their head for even a short time. This means that it is very difficult for them to form new long-term memories, because if the information doesn't get into the short-term store in the first place, it can't then be transferred into long-term storage.

People with dementia still have information in their long-term memory store, though slowly this is lost with the disease. Imagine that the long-term memory system of the brain is a tall, narrow storage box with the opening at the top. Our earliest childhood memories are stored at the bottom of the box and our most recent memories are at the top. As the brain is eroded by dementia, the storage box deteriorates from the top down, so memories that were stored most recently are lost first. The person then sometimes thinks that older memories are actually recent memories of current events and people. This is why people with severe dementia often seem to be living in the past and remember the details of things that happened decades ago very clearly, but can't remember what they had for lunch today. The person with dementia may also have trouble accessing the information in their long-term store. This is similar to the situation when the internet stops working and we can't access our files stored online. The information is still there, we just can't get to it, and later on the system may work again and we can get the information again.

Having missing information from their long-term memory means that people with moderate to severe dementia are often operating in a situation or place they can't remember. They can't remember the person, even if they have interacted with them before, and have to figure out who the person is, whether he is trustworthy and how to relate to him. This may be complicated if the stranger seems to know the person with dementia, and the person with dementia might have to pretend to know them in order to be polite. The person with dementia might not remember a place, even if they have been there many times, and will have to figure out where things are located, such as the toilet. Having to figure things out all the time can be very tiring. When we travel or start a new job, most of us find it more mentally tiring than a routine day at work or home, because in these situations we have to process so much more new information relating to people and places.

We usually think of memory as retrospective, or relating to the past. However there is one form of memory that relates to future events. This is called prospective memory, and is the memory for things that we need to do in the future, for instance remembering to go to the doctor at 9 a.m. on Tuesday, or remembering to check the cake after it's been in the oven for an hour. People with dementia have difficulties with prospective memory, meaning that they find it hard to remember to do at the right time things that they want to do or have agreed to in the past. Prospective-memory difficulties lead to pots on the stove boiling dry and not being ready on time.

PRACTICAL TIPS

Use memory aids to help with short-term memory difficulties: lists, notebooks, diaries and calendars. Electronic devices such as smart phones can help with prospective memory if an alarm is set with a reminder to do things at certain times. Write notes and leave them where they will be seen at the right time (e.g. place a note at the front door for reminders when leaving the house — 'Have you got your keys, phone and wallet?'). Have a routine for things so that the person with dementia doesn't have to rely on memory as much. Program important phone numbers into your phone.

Having difficulties with short-term memory means that it is easier to lose track of what day and time it is. Put clocks in every room. Have a calendar in a prominent place, make a note of the date, day and month in the morning, mark off the day each evening.

Carers need to be aware of and compensate for the poor short-term memory of people with dementia. Give instructions one sentence at a time, or a phrase at a time, or even a word at a time.

Try to guess at what stage in their past the person with dementia believes they are living. For some people with dementia there is a gradual shift into the past, for others the shift is more pronounced. Do they think they are aged in their eighties with three grandchildren? Or do they believe that they are aged in their fifties and working? Or do they think that they are in their twenties with young children? Talking with the person with dementia in a way that is consistent with their beliefs will be less confusing for them. Giving him or her activities that fit within their beliefs will also be more meaningful for them. For instance, a gentleman who believes he still works may find it meaningful to get 'dressed' for the office, and sit at a table and sort cards on a topic relating to his past employment. A woman who thinks she has young children may enjoy folding children's clothes or cloth nappies, or looking after a baby doll.

The poor short-term memory of people with dementia means that they forget the pleasure and fun they shared with you. If it is important to you that they remember some of the things you do together, take photos of you doing things together and things that you have seen and display these in a place where the person will see them (the mantelpiece, fridge or bedside table). This will help them relive the experience (if not the memory).

When talking with people with dementia, instead of asking questions about recent events, comment on things that you can both see, smell, hear or taste at that time. Discuss the people, animals and things in nature that you experience around you. There is no point in arguing with a person with dementia on a point relating to their memory; if he doesn't remember that you visited yesterday or that you told him that information 5 minutes ago, insisting that you did won't convince him.

Difficulties with memory mean that people with dementia are constantly re-creating their past using the faded memories they have and clues from the present. Imagine waking up and not remembering where you are or how you got there. You'd try to figure out what happened based on your last memory (e.g. I was buying bananas in the fruit shop) and clues from the present (I'm lying down and there is a woman who is in some sort of uniform; maybe she is a nurse?). For people with dementia, it may be difficult to piece together an accurate understanding of their current situation because their 'recent' memory may be from quite far in the past. People with dementia sometimes make up an imaginary explanation to compensate for their loss of memory. We call this confabulation. Giving the person with dementia information in their environment about the present may help them understand their current situation. Some nursing homes encourage residents to furnish their room with familiar objects and furniture — these clues can help the person with dementia think of the care facility as the place where they live.

DIFFICULTIES WITH ATTENTION

Babies find the world endlessly fascinating to the point of being overstimulating. Everything is new and interesting and they are easily distracted by the next new, noisy, bright or moving thing. Being able to focus our attention on one thing at a time is an ability that we develop. Being able to concentrate in this way is useful in getting things done. We see people working intently on their laptops at cafés, tuning out with their mind the hustle and bustle around them. Tuning or blocking out distractions is part of focusing attention. We can tune or block out distractions physically, such as when we close our eyes or cover our ears when we're trying to think.

People with dementia lose their ability to focus their attention. They find it especially difficult to cope in noisy situations with many people. When sharing activities with people with dementia, it helps them if we can take away potential distractions so that they don't have to spend mental energy screening out that information. This could mean switching off the radio or television, taking them into a quiet room without other people, and removing things unrelated to the activity. When talking to the person with dementia, give them one piece of information at a time, and give them time to take it in before presenting the next piece. For people with severe dementia, it can be confusing to have two people visiting or taking care of them. It may be easier for them to focus their attention on one person at a time. If a second person is helping with personal care, they can be an extra set of hands as unobtrusively as possible.

People with dementia cannot concentrate for as long as other adults, since for them focusing attention takes much more mental energy. We need to watch for signs that the person is no longer interested in an activity or that they are tiring. Such signs could be that they stop looking at the activity or person and start looking away, they stop participating, or they say they want to stop. In mild dementia, they may be able to participate intensely for 45 minutes to an hour. In more moderate dementia, about half an hour, and in severe dementia 5 to 15 minutes might be all they can manage.

PRACTICAL TIPS

Noisy group situations can be difficult to cope with because the person needs to spend energy blocking out the distractions. In noisy situations, give the person a break in a quiet place. If you're in a situation where it is difficult to leave the group (e.g. at a family weekend together), the person might enjoy listening to music they like through headphones, just so they can stop concentrating for a while.

DIFFICULTIES WITH INITIATION

To initiate means to take the first step to start something. We need to think about wanting to do something and then start the process of doing it. Initiation is critical to even simple activities such as getting dressed, having something to eat or having a conversation. The only common activity that doesn't necessarily require initiation is sleeping; sometimes we just drift off to sleep without meaning to. Initiation is also needed for more complicated activities such as going out to the shops, paying a bill or making a meal.

Apathy is almost universal in people with dementia. They lose their ability to initiate, which means that they lose their get up and go, their 'on–off' switch gets stuck on 'off'. They may not think of getting dressed and instead stay in their pyjamas all day. They mean to pay a bill but do not get around to doing it. We need to flick 'on' the activity switch for them. Some people with dementia might just need help to initiate the start of an activity, while others might need help initiating each step of that activity. We can do this by asking them to start doing things. Alternatively, we can leave out objects that may prompt them to start something. Laying out their clothes on their bed may encourage a person with dementia to get dressed. Putting the bill on the dining-room table with a note saying 'I am now due, please pay me' may prompt the person with dementia to pay the bill.

DIFFICULTIES WITH DECISION MAKING, PROBLEM SOLVING AND PLANNING

Decision making, problem solving and planning are more complex types of thinking that develop later in childhood. Decision making involves choosing between two or more alternatives by considering the possible consequences of those choices. Problem solving involves developing possible solutions for a problem and then deciding between those possible solutions. Planning involves working out the steps towards a goal then using problem-solving and decision-making strategies for each step. Even as adults, decision making, planning and problem solving can be difficult and require a lot of mental effort and energy.

The principle of 'last in, first out' of the brain of a person with dementia that I described in relation to memory also applies to decision making, problem solving and planning. Relatively early in the disease, people with dementia lose the ability to first plan and problem solve, and then the ability to make complex decisions.

Decision making, problem solving and planning all involve working with thoughts or abstract ideas rather than real-life objects. When we make decisions, we draw on our memories of past experiences to imagine the future consequences of each alternative, and choose the most appealing consequence. When we problem solve, we create in our minds a range of possible solutions. People with dementia have more difficulty with abstract thought, with using logic to imagine consequences and create solutions within the parameters of the problem.

We usually need to do most of the planning and problem solving for people with dementia. However, as much as possible we should involve them in decision making. Freedom of choice is something that is important for us as humans to have. For people with moderate to severe dementia, you may need to present the alternatives visually to make the decision easier — for instance, showing them the packages of chicken and sausage from the fridge when asking what they'd like to eat, or showing them a photograph of a beach or a park when asking where they would like to go.

PRACTICAL TIPS

There are often many pieces of information to consider in decision making, problem solving and planning. For simpler decisions we usually keep all the information about the possible choices and consequences in our short-term memory. When helping people with dementia make decisions, write down the options and pros and cons of each as you discuss them. If possible, use pictures to communicate the options (e.g. of the different people you're talking about visiting, or of the places you're talking about going to). 'Talking Mats' is a picture-based tool to help people with dementia and carers make decisions together (see 'Further resources' on p. 230).

If you find that the person with dementia is taking longer than you would like to make everyday decisions, such as what clothes to wear or what to put in their sandwich, then simplify those decisions. For instance, work with them to match their clothes into sets and hang these together so they can just take a set out of the cupboard each morning. Put all the sandwich ingredients for a sandwich that they like in the one spot in the fridge, even the things that don't need to be refrigerated, so they can just get them out and make the sandwich.

DIFFICULTIES WITH SPEECH AND COMPREHENSION

Conversations are important ways of interacting with other people. In order to understand what someone else is saying we have to process the sounds the other person makes and interpret the meaning of the words within the sentence. To reply, we decide what idea we want to express, find the right words and the right order for the words, and then say them aloud.

Any (and many) of these steps can go wrong for a person with dementia. Usually, they start with having trouble expressing themselves, with finding the right words and putting them into a sentence. Their poor memory means that they find it hard to follow complex stories and even long sentences. They may lose their understanding of the meanings of words, though usually keep their ability to read tone and body language.

DIFFICULTIES WITH PERCEPTION

As children, we are taught that we see with our eyes, hear with our ears, smell with our nose, taste with our tongue and feel through our skin. This isn't entirely accurate. Our sensory organs are the receptors; information they collect is sent to the brain, which processes and interprets the information. We actually see, hear, smell, taste and feel with our brains as much as our sensory organs. For example, our brain interprets the pattern of light hitting our retina as a seagull, the pattern of vibrations hitting our eardrums as the sound of waves crashing, and the chemicals entering our nose as the smell of the seaside.

The ability of people with dementia to interpret visual information changes as their brain deteriorates, even if their eyesight is fine. They sometimes do not 'see' objects that are right in front of them. This may be because they do not recognize the object for what it is because it does not match their schema or mental template of what that object should look like. An extreme example is someone whose schema of a telephone is from the 1970s — they would therefore not recognize a mobile phone as being a telephone. Alternatively, they may have an incorrect memory of what the object should look like: for instance it is difficult to find a book when you think the cover is red but it is actually white.

People with dementia also lose their ability to detect and distinguish smells, and this happens early in the course of dementia. Since smell contributes a great deal to how we perceive flavour, they also have impaired ability to taste. This may result in changes to their appetite or the food they like.

If the person with dementia seems to have difficulty with seeing things, and this is not due to a problem with their eyesight, then modify their environment to help them see important objects. Reduce visual clutter so the person doesn't have to use their attention to block out irrelevant objects. Aim for maximum contrast between the things you want them to notice and their background. Text should be large (32-point minimum) and be black on white, or white on black. Food should be contrasting in colour to the plate — a white sandwich or white fish and mashed potato on a white plate on a white tablecloth is less obvious than when placed on a blue plate. Similarly, you could place a white doily between a dark wallet and dark wood table to make the wallet more obvious. If the person is having trouble finding the toilet, then getting a contrasting toilet seat may help.

CHANGES IN PERSONALITY, AND DIFFICULTIES CONTROLLING FEELINGS

Personality, character, temperament — these all describe our individual and unique ways of behaving, feeling and thinking. We think that our personality develops through a combination of our genetic disposition (for example, a disposition to be extroverted or introverted) and our upbringing and experiences through life. A naturally extroverted person could end up being bossy and overbearing, or motivating and outgoing. A naturally introverted person could end up being shy and retiring, or quietly confident.

There is no clear pattern in how personality changes as a result of dementia, however a change in personality is often one of the early symptoms of the condition. Some people with dementia seem to have their personality characteristics exaggerated. Someone who had a short fuse gets angry even more quickly, someone who was a worrier is even more anxious. However, some people with dementia seem to have their personality traits softened. Someone who used to be grumpy becomes more easygoing, someone who was outgoing is more passive.

Exaggerated personality may develop because the person's ability to judge the appropriateness of an action has deteriorated. Most of us have the ability to moderate or censor our actions, so we stop and decide whether a particular action is a good idea before doing it. When we are feeling angry this ability to self-censor stops us from punching the person we are angry with or throwing the teapot out the window because we may be arrested for assault or might smash the teapot. Some people with dementia will act more impulsively and behave according to their personality with less consideration of the consequences. The same part of the brain that decides whether a particular action is a good idea, the frontal lobe, also helps us control our feelings. This is an ability we (well, most of us anyway) develop in early adulthood. Toddlers and teenagers sometimes seem to have very labile, rapidly fluctuating and unreasonable emotional reactions because this area of the brain isn't fully developed. Some people with dementia act this way too, because of deteriorations in the frontal lobe.

Dampened personalities in people with dementia may occur because the areas of the brain where personality is 'stored' have been damaged, or because they lack the initiative to behave or react the way they previously did.

DIFFICULTIES WITH MOVEMENT

Dementia affects speed, coordination, balance and strength because these abilities are controlled by the brain. This means that people with dementia are not as agile as they were previously, are more likely to fall and can have poorer fine motor skills. When planning activities, their current physical abilities should be taken into account. Physical activities that they could previously manage may be more difficult now: they might not be able to walk as far, might not be as comfortable on uneven ground and could tire more easily.

EQUATING PEOPLE WITH DEMENTIA AND CHILDREN

I have discussed how the deterioration of mental abilities with dementia mirrors the development of these same abilities in children. It can be useful to think of people with mild dementia who can travel independently as being similar to children aged eight to twelve years, people with moderate dementia who are independent in their self-care as being similar to children aged five to seven years, people with moderately severe dementia who may need prompting but can dress and shower themselves as being similar to children aged three to five years, and those with severe dementia who need physical help with self-care as being similar to children aged younger than two. The similarities can help you think about what the person can do independently, including the decisions about their life and safety that they can make independently, and the kind of activities they might do and enjoy.

However, this does not mean we should treat people with dementia the way that we treat children. There are some important differences between people with dementia and children that we should be aware of:

- Children's brains are in a period of growth and development. This drives them to carefully observe and rapidly absorb and process knowledge about the world. In contrast, the brains of people with dementia are declining and deteriorating and while they can still learn new things, they do so at a slower rate than children. They also have a poorer and slower ability to observe and process the world.
- People with dementia have lived long lives as adults, and as such should be accorded the respect that older adults deserve.
- In general, children have much more initiative and enthusiasm than people with dementia. They are geared to play and learn! People with dementia tend to be apathetic and increasingly lose confidence in their abilities.

- Children generally have good hearing and vision, and good (or improving) coordination, balance and fine motor skills. These often have declined in people with dementia.
- Children have a small bank of knowledge and experiences of the world. People with dementia have an extensive bank of knowledge and life experiences, though these memories may become increasingly difficult to access.

It may be helpful to think about these similarities between persons with dementia and young children:

- They both have difficulties at times expressing what they want, and sometimes do not really know what is wrong themselves. As a consequence they can act out rather than speak out when something is wrong.
- They both have a limited ability to concentrate for long periods.
- They both learn better by doing and copying rather than by listening to or reading instructions (as do many adults!).
- They rely on body language much more than the content of the words.

THEORY OF UNMET NEEDS AND BEHAVIOURAL AND PSYCHOLOGICAL SYMPTOMS OF DEMENTIA

There is a theory that suggests many of the symptoms of dementia (such as agitation, aggression, pacing, yelling, arguing and depression) arise because people with dementia have needs that are not being met. They may feel disturbed or uncomfortable but do not recognize the reason for these feelings, or they may not be able to express what is wrong. Young children often act in difficult ways because of similar reasons. Research has shown that identifying and attending to these needs of people with dementia decreases these behaviours that for carers can often be distressing and difficult to cope with. Research has also shown that doing activities can decrease these behaviours. These activities seem to be more successful in decreasing behaviours when they are tailored to the person with dementia.

The unmet needs of people with dementia generally fall into three areas.

1. Physical health — they might be in pain, feel too hot or too cold, feel unwell, hungry, thirsty or need to use the toilet.

2. Stimulation — they may feel overstimulated and not be able to cope with a situation that is too noisy or where there are too many people; or they may be understimulated and feel bored or unoccupied, and have excess energy.

3. Company — they may want someone to be with for company, reassurance and companionship.

What the science tells us

Dementia is the umbrella term for a group of neurodegenerative conditions in which brain deterioration causes the symptoms of dementia. Different types of dementia affect the brain differently, which is why they produce different symptoms. Most types of dementia are defined by the causes of the brain deterioration, but some are defined by the location of the deterioration. Four common types of dementia are described below; there are many others.

The changes in the brain associated with Alzheimer's disease, neuritic plaques and neurofibrillary tangles tend to damage neuronal material in the hippocampus first. The hippocampus helps with the formation of new memories. That is why short-term memory loss is one of the early symptoms in people with Alzheimer's disease. The hippocampus also deteriorates as part of normal brain ageing, so our short-term memory ability also deteriorates as we grow older, which makes it difficult to distinguish the early symptoms of Alzheimer's disease from normal ageing.

Another change in the brain of people with Alzheimer's disease is general atrophy or shrinking of the brain, caused by death of the brain cells, and loss of the connection between the cells. The brain of someone with Alzheimer's disease shrinks up to three times faster than the brain of an older person without the condition. This means that the whole brain of the person with Alzheimer's disease starts working less effectively, it works more slowly and inconsistently and sometimes does not succeed in its tasks. The cognitive decline in Alzheimer's can be thought of as a gentle slope, starting off mildly and with loss of ability decreasing slowly and increasingly across time.

Vascular dementia is caused by large, small or very small strokes in the brain. The strokes or transient ischemic attacks might be so mild that the person might not realize they have had a stroke. The strokes result in the death of cells in one large area or multiple small areas of the brain. The symptoms will depend on which brain areas have been affected. This is similar to people who have a stroke that affects them physically on only one side of their body. People with vascular dementia can have a range of different symptoms and can perform poorly on one aspect of thinking yet still perform well in other aspects. The cognitive decline in vascular dementia is more like downward steps, with each step corresponding to a new stroke or mini stroke in the brain.

In fronto-temporal dementia the frontal and temporal lobes deteriorate much more than the rest of the brain. This can be caused by a variety of issues. The frontal lobe is the part of the brain responsible for problem solving, planning and modifying behaviour. So people with fronto-temporal dementia tend to have poor impulse control, poor planning and poor problem-solving skills. The temporal lobe includes the hippocampus and other brain areas involved in memory formation, consolidation and retrieval, so memory is affected depending on how much the temporal lobe is affected.

Dementia with Lewy bodies (or Lewy body dementia) is named after the Lewy bodies that develop in brain cells. Lewy bodies are clumps of alpha-synuclein and ubiquitin proteins, and they are thought to cause the death of brain cells. People with Lewy body dementia tend to have variable mental abilities, so sometimes they seem almost normal and at other times they are confused and disoriented. They often have visual hallucinations or delusions, meaning that they see things that are not really there or believe things to be true that are not. They also often have a tremor or stiffness in their movements.

With the exception of vascular dementia, the causes of the other common forms of dementia are not known. We know, however, about a range of factors that can decrease the risk of developing any form of dementia, such as looking after our hearts and staying within the recommended guidelines for cholesterol, blood pressure and weight; eating a healthy diet; engaging in regular physical exercise and regular mental exercise; not smoking or drinking to excess; and avoiding brain injury.

We used to believe that we were born with a set number of brain cells, called neurons. It was thought that throughout life we gradually lost these neurons. Then scientists discovered that the brain grows new neurons, and that the environment affects the rate of growth and survival of these new neurons. In mouse models of Alzheimer's disease, new neurons continue to grow, and growth rates can be stimulated through physical, mental and social activity.

IDENTIFYING THE COGNITIVE ABILITIES OF THE PERSON WITH DEMENTIA

We need to understand the cognitive abilities of the people with dementia we care for so that we can modify the activities to ensure they can do them successfully. Table 1 (p. 32) is intended to help you identify the current thinking abilities of the person with dementia you care for. The table focuses on abilities that will affect what activities you do with them, and how you present them. It is not intended to replace a formal cognitive or neuropsychological assessment to diagnose dementia, or to assess change in cognitive abilities. Rather it is intended to help carers figure out what the person with dementia may be able to do, and also may help show relative strengths and weaknesses of the person with dementia.

Those of us who get to know people with dementia after they have developed dementia find it easier to accept and work with the strengths and personality of the person as we find them, since we did not know them beforehand. Carers who have known the person from before the onset of dementia sometimes spend emotional energy noticing and worrying about the mental abilities that have deteriorated and remembering the person in their prime. While these memories are important, it can be more productive to focus on the person's current strengths and on how to maximize their current abilities.

It is sometimes very difficult to judge what a person with dementia can do. As a psychologist, I'm often surprised at their abilities when I test a person — which can be much worse or much better than I expect, or can be unexpectedly good in one aspect of thinking or memory. I tend to expect that people with dementia with good social skills will also have good mental abilities, but social skills and mental abilities do not always correspond. Alzheimer's dementia is the most common form of the disease and so most professionals have a 'prototype' of dementia that is most similar to Alzheimer's disease, with memory problems being the predominant early complaint. Other types of dementia often are quite different. For instance, someone with vascular dementia may have relatively good short-term memory but very poor judgment. Family and professional carers often underestimate or overestimate the abilities of a person with dementia.

The only way to know what a person with dementia can do is to be observant, and to consider each ability individually. You may need to make these observations before completing the tables. You may be surprised at what the person you care for can still do, and might realize that you've been doing too much for him or her. Or you may be surprised at how little they can do, and reflect that they have been understanding less of what is going on than you thought or may need more supervision than you have been giving.

It may be useful to review the table and update your answers if the person with dementia's condition changes.

Table 1: Assessing current thinking abilities

Record as best you can the thinking abilities of the person with dementia you care for, by circling the most appropriate description.   Date:_____

	Typical dementia stage (rough guide, and people can have thinking abilities across different stages)			
	Mild dementia	Mild to moderate dementia	Moderate to severe dementia	Severe dementia
Short-term memory	Can sometimes remember things from the week before or better	Can sometimes remember things from the day before	Can sometimes remember events from earlier that day	Hardly ever remembers recent events
Long-term memory *Seems to talk most about memories from_____ period in life*	Remembers things well from middle age	Remembers things well from young adulthood	Remembers things from childhood, or little memory of past	Hardly ever seems to remember the past
Goal direction	Can remember the goal of most activities and complete steps to achieve goal	Can remember the goals of familiar activities and with help can complete steps to achieve goal	Can sometimes remember the goal of familiar activities, and can complete simple steps	Does not seem to remember or understand most familiar activities
Attention	Can sometimes concentrate for 30–60 minutes	Can sometimes concentrate for 15–30 minutes	Can sometimes concentrate for up to 15 minutes	Can sometimes concentrate for up to 5 minutes
Decision making	Can choose from multiple options that are named but not shown	Can choose from multiple options that are shown	Can choose from two options that are shown	Does not usually make choices when offered

	Typical dementia stage (rough guide, and people can have thinking abilities across different stages)			
	Mild dementia	Mild to moderate dementia	Moderate to severe dementia	Severe dementia
Communicating	Speaks using sentences, though may have difficulty finding the right words	Speaks using short phrases	Communicates using single words or through body language	Communicates through body language only
Understanding	Can follow a conversation of several sentences in a row	Can follow a conversation of one sentence at a time	Can follow a conversation using simple phrases and body language	Can understand single words (e.g. their name) and body language
Coordination abilities	Has good hand–eye coordination and can manipulate objects in complex sequences (e.g. tying a shoe lace)	Has good hand–eye coordination and can manipulate objects in complex sequences	Has reasonable hand–eye coordination and can manipulate objects in simple sequences	Has difficulty controlling hands and manipulating objects

Additionally, take note of and record the following information (particularly if this information is being completed by professional care staff, or will be shared with professional care staff):

Right handed		Left handed
Hearing good both ears		Hearing poor both ears
Hearing better right ear		Hearing better left ear
Sight good both eyes		Sight poor both eyes
Sight better right eye		Sight better left eye

2

TAKING A LIFE HISTORY

The key to success in giving an activity to a person with dementia is that it has to be *engaging*. By engaging I mean interesting, pleasing, attractive, fascinating, entertaining, captivating, agreeable or likable. The person with dementia has to want to start doing it and keep doing it. Preferably the activity will be actively engaging, so instead of just passively watching the activity the person will want to actively take part. Watching something activates some brain areas; however, actually participating activates more brain areas more strongly.

An activity is more likely to be engaging for someone with dementia if it is:

- meaningful — of interest or value to the person
- achievable — at a level at which they can successfully participate in or complete it.

Along with your understanding of their current abilities, another important tool in choosing appropriate activities for the person you care for is knowledge of their life history. This is the focus of this chapter.

THE STEPS TO CHOOSING APPROPRIATE ACTIVITIES

Choosing appropriate activities for a person with dementia is an art, not a science. The process is somewhat trial and error; some activities you try will be enthusiastically and positively received, others will be rejected and others will simply be met with disinterest. Each reaction, positive or negative, will give you information that will increase the likelihood of success for the next activity you try.

Here are the basic steps.

1. Identify the person's current abilities (you already did this in Chapter 1). This information will help you tailor activities so that they are achievable by the person with dementia.

2. Find out about the person's life history (this is the topic of this chapter). This information will help you select or tailor activities so that they are meaningful to the person.

3. Use the information gathered in steps 1 and 2 to brainstorm ideas for how to tailor activities for the person with dementia. This is the topic of Chapter 3, however the remaining chapters all give ideas for selecting and tailoring different types of activities.

4. Trial each activity and reflect, modify and amend it where needed.

COMPONENTS OF A LIFE HISTORY

In order to maximize the enjoyment and engagement of the person with dementia, we start by choosing topics or activities that they used to enjoy in the past or that are related to their life in some way.

If you know the person well, you may already know their social history; nonetheless it is helpful to write this information down and reflect on it in preparation for brainstorming activities that they may enjoy. If you don't know the person with dementia well, try to ask them about their social history, even if they cannot converse with you fluently or answer all your questions. Interview or consult with a family member or friend who knows the person, too, to get as much information as you can. There is a worksheet on page 39 that will help you document this information.

Here are important components of most people's life histories, which help in planning activities to do with them.

Places of significance (one or two)

Where were they born? Where did they spend their childhood? Where did they live? Are there any places that are special to them and why?

The 'culture' the person grew up in and lived in may be an important topic for them. Information about culture may also help others understand the lens through which the person is interpreting their current surroundings. For instance, if the person grew up during wartime in a culture of deprivation and suspicion, the person may be suspicious of authority figures, ultra-protective of their possessions and constantly worried about the safety of their family.

People of significance

Who are or were the important people in their life? Most often this is a spouse and children, but it could also be a parent, or best friend or other relative. What was the person with dementia's relationship with the person like, and what is the relationship currently like?

Activities of significance

What did the person do for a job? What did the person do in their spare time? Were there any things the person was particularly passionate about? Activities can be anything at all that the person was interested in, ranging from an individual hobby, something they did around the house, a group activity (church, Rotary) or even something that they only did actively for a little while but continued to be interested in (e.g. played cricket during adolescence and followed the game throughout life).

Identify activities that the person with dementia currently enjoys doing. These could be small things such as going for a walk or listening to music. We need to keep doing these things with them, and you may be able to build on and extend these activities.

Events of significance

Were there any events (negative or positive) the person experienced that were important to them? These could have been life-changing activities such as fighting in a war, living through an earthquake or having a child. These could also include memorable events such as watching a Melbourne Cup race live, meeting the prime minister or competing for their country. If the event is negative and the person didn't like talking about it, then it is particularly important to document this and make sure to avoid this topic.

Personal recreation preferences

Did they like to do things quietly by themselves, or did they like doing things in groups? When in groups, did they like to be the organizer, or participate but not be the centre of attention? Did they enjoy being with people they knew well or did they like meeting new people? How did they like to 'play'?

What is missing?

What is missing from the person's life? Is it company, or meaning, or employment or a feeling of being valued and important? What roles did they have previously that were important to them that they have lost?

If there are many people involved in the care of the person with dementia, some of whom may not know the person well, it may also be useful to create an 'all about me' sheet with the key information written down and including photos if possible so that it is easy to share this information with any new carers. There are also books and templates that Dementia Australia has published that can be used to help record information for carers (see 'Further resources' p. 230).

PRACTICAL TIPS

Here are some questions to ask the person with dementia which may give you ideas for enriching their life.

- Imagine what a great day for you would be. What would you do or talk about? Who would you be with? Where would you be? What would you eat and drink?

- Are there any things you have always wanted to do but haven't managed to yet? This may be something big, like travelling to Europe, or something small, like going fishing or making bread.
- Who are the people you want to spend time with? This might include people you see often and others you see less often or have lost touch with. Could you get in touch with lost friends? Can you use telephone, email, Skype or letters to communicate?
- What do you like doing now that you would like to keep doing?

Table 2: Life history worksheet for activity planning

Write life history information in this column	Brainstorm possible activities in this column (will be discussed in Chapter 3)
Places of significance	
People of significance	
Activities of significance (including present activities)	
Events of significance	
Personal recreation preferences	
What is missing?	

CASE STUDIES

Throughout the book we will look at the lives of four people living with dementia: Joy, Antonio, Ruth and Brian. We will learn more about their stories and their interactions with their carers through the rest of this book. Let's start by taking a look at each of their life stories along with the table assessing each person's current thinking abilities (see Table 1 on p. 32).

Case study

Joy

Joy has mild Alzheimer's disease and lives at home with her husband.

1. Places of significance

Joy was born in Surry Hills in Sydney and has lived there all her life. For her honeymoon, her husband took her to England and France, places for which she has a special fondness. They would take overseas trips every two or three years, though she appears to remember these less clearly.

2. People of significance

Joy and Bernie married relatively late, in their thirties, and did not have any children. Bernie ran an accounting business and until lately was active with their local Probus club. They are not close to any family, and Bernie says that while Joy had lots of friends they seem to have fallen away since she developed dementia and her conversation and behaviour changed. She only goes with Bernie to Probus club events now, and does not talk much at those.

3. Activities of significance

Joy worked in retail, in fashion boutiques, for many years. She then worked casually as an extra in film and television, and continued to do this work into her late sixties. She said she enjoyed meeting people in show business. While describing herself as not being a good cook, Joy said she liked having people over, and Bernie says she was quite the hostess. Joy continues to take pride in her appearance and always puts on lipstick and powder before going out.

4. Events of significance

According to Joy, the most important event in her life was her marriage to Bernie and their honeymoon.

5. Personal recreation preference

Bernie describes Joy as extroverted and someone who liked to make people happy. She liked being with others rather than being alone; this is more so since she developed dementia.

6. What is missing?

Joy says that she is happy with her lovely husband and home and that there is nothing missing in her life. Bernie says, however, that Joy misses having other women to talk to.

Here is the table for Joy, detailing her current thinking abilities. We can see that Joy's abilities match a typical pattern for Alzheimer's dementia. She has slight difficulties but has the cognitive abilities to participate in many different activities.

| | Typical dementia stage (rough guide, and people can have thinking abilities across different stages) | | | |
	Mild dementia	Mild to moderate dementia	Moderate to severe dementia	Severe dementia
Short-term memory	Can sometimes remember things from the week before or better	Can sometimes remember things from the day before	Can sometimes remember events from earlier that day	Hardly ever remembers recent events
Long-term memory *Seems to talk most about memories from_____ period in life*	Remembers things well from middle age	Remembers things well from young adulthood	Remembers things from childhood, or little memory of past	Hardly ever seems to remember the past
Goal direction	Can remember the goal of most activities and complete steps to achieve goal	Can remember the goals of familiar activities and with help can complete steps to achieve goal	Can sometimes remember the goal of familiar activities, and can complete simple steps	Does not seem to remember or understand most familiar activities
Attention	Can sometimes concentrate for 30–60 minutes	Can sometimes concentrate for 15–30 minutes	Can sometimes concentrate for up to 15 minutes	Can sometimes concentrate for up to 5 minutes

	Typical dementia stage (rough guide, and people can have thinking abilities across different stages)			
	Mild dementia	Mild to moderate dementia	Moderate to severe dementia	Severe dementia
Decision making	Can choose from multiple options that are named but not shown	Can choose from multiple options that are shown	Can choose from two options that are shown	Does not usually make choices when offered
Communicating	Speaks using sentences, though may have difficulty finding the right words	Speaks using short phrases	Communicates using single words or through body language	Communicates through body language only
Understanding	Can follow a conversation of several sentences in a row	Can follow a conversation of one sentence at a time	Can follow a conversation using simple phrases and body language	Can understand single words (e.g. their name) and body language
Coordination abilities	Has good hand–eye coordination and can manipulate objects in complex sequences (e.g. tying a shoe lace)	Has good hand–eye coordination and can manipulate objects in complex sequences	Has reasonable hand–eye coordination and can manipulate objects in simple sequences	Has difficulty controlling hands and manipulating objects

Case study

Antonio

Antonio has mild to moderate vascular dementia and lives at home with his wife, Maria.

1. Places of significance

Antonio was born in Sicily, Italy. He migrated to Australia after World War II with his brother, Francesco. After working on a farm for five years, he started a convenience store in Brunswick, Melbourne. He has lived in South Melbourne since.

2. People of significance

Antonio's wife, Maria, is twenty years his junior. They were introduced through family in Italy and corresponded by mail before Antonio returned to Italy to court her. Maria agreed to marry him and came to Australia to be wed the next year. They had two children, a boy, Antonio Jr, and a girl, Sofia. Antonio was close to his older brother, Francesco, however Francesco also has dementia and now lives in a nursing home.

3. Activities of significance

Antonio worked hard in his convenience store business, which at its peak had ten employees. He was also active with the Brunswick Juventus Soccer Club, and in its heyday and afterwards would regularly attend games and support fundraising events. Currently he does very little: he waters the plants and enjoys his food.

4. Events of significance

Antonio talks about his marriage to Maria and the birth of his children as being important events in his life. Another significant event was having to close his convenience store and retire in the mid 1990s because financially it was more profitable to sell to developers, who wanted to renovate the building and turn it into housing. Maria reports that in 1985 Brunswick Juventus won the national soccer league, which was also an important time for Antonio.

5. Personal recreation preference

Maria describes Antonio as having been a sociable but private man. He knew everyone in the neighbourhood but didn't take many people into his inner circle except for his brother and family.

6. What is missing?

Maria says that Antonio misses having a purpose in his life. He also has lost confidence in what he knows and in being able to make decisions for his family.

Here is the table for Antonio. He has more difficulties with attention and concentration and may need to be more supported in tasks requiring these skills.

| | Typical dementia stage (rough guide, and people can have thinking abilities across different stages) | | | |
	Mild dementia	Mild to moderate dementia	Moderate to severe dementia	Severe dementia
Short-term memory	Can sometimes remember things from the week before or better	Can sometimes remember things from the day before	Can sometimes remember events from earlier that day	Hardly ever remembers recent events
Long-term memory *Seems to talk most about memories from_____ period in life*	Remembers things well from middle age	Remembers things well from young adulthood	Remembers things from childhood, or little memory of past	Hardly ever seems to remember the past
Goal direction	Can remember the goal of most activities and complete steps to achieve goal	Can remember the goals of familiar activities and with help can complete steps to achieve goal	Can sometimes remember the goal of familiar activities, and can complete simple steps	Does not seem to remember or understand most familiar activities
Attention	Can sometimes concentrate for 30–60 minutes	Can sometimes concentrate for 15–30 minutes	Can sometimes concentrate for up to 15 minutes	Can sometimes concentrate for up to 5 minutes
Decision making	Can choose from multiple options that are named but not shown	Can choose from multiple options that are shown	Can choose from two options that are shown	Does not usually make choices when offered

	Typical dementia stage (rough guide, and people can have thinking abilities across different stages)			
	Mild dementia	Mild to moderate dementia	Moderate to severe dementia	Severe dementia
Communicating	Speaks using sentences, though may have difficulty finding the right words	Speaks using short phrases	Communicates using single words or through body language	Communicates through body language only
Understanding	Can follow a conversation of several sentences in a row	Can follow a conversation of one sentence at a time	Can follow a conversation using simple phrases and body language	Can understand single words (e.g. their name) and body language
Coordination abilities	Has good hand–eye coordination and can manipulate objects in complex sequences (e.g. tying a shoe lace)	Has good hand–eye coordination and can manipulate objects in complex sequences	Has reasonable hand–eye coordination and can manipulate objects in simple sequences	Has difficulty controlling hands and manipulating objects

Case study

Ruth

Ruth has moderate mixed vascular dementia and Alzheimer's disease. She lives in a nursing home.

1. Places of significance

Ruth was born in Bath, England, and migrated with her husband and three daughters to Australia in her thirties. They lived in Brisbane and Adelaide before retiring to the Adelaide Hills.

2. People of significance

Ruth's three daughters are Jane, Julie and Hannah. Julie and Hannah both live in Adelaide, Jane lives in England. She has several grandchildren, and was particularly close to Jade and Jordan, whom she would often look after. Ruth's husband passed away when the girls were teenagers and Ruth never remarried. Ruth's best friend is Helena. She used to have lunch once a month in Adelaide with a group of former colleagues from the hospital where she worked for many years.

3. Activities of significance

Ruth worked as a nurse her whole life, first in the maternity ward, then in the general wards. When her husband died, she often worked night shifts so she could be home during the day for the girls. She took up knitting and crochet when she worked night shift as she said it helped her pass the quiet times. Later she was active in the hospital's fundraising committee and she donated many handmade items for sale in hospital fundraisers. Ruth no longer undertakes any activities.

4. Events of significance

Ruth's daughter Hannah describes Ruth as being proud that all her three daughters graduated from university, and that after her last daughter graduated Ruth said she had done her job.

5. Personal recreation preference

Hannah describes Ruth as being sociable but quiet. 'She spent her life caring for others,' says Hannah.

6. What is missing?

Hannah and Julie both talk about Ruth losing confidence and not having anything to do any more. They say she no longer has a role in life because she can't help people any more.

Here is the table for Ruth. She has relatively good communication abilities, relative to her memory and attention.

| | Typical dementia stage (rough guide, and people can have thinking abilities across different stages) | | | |
	Mild dementia	Mild to moderate dementia	Moderate to severe dementia	Severe dementia
Short-term memory	Can sometimes remember things from the week before or better	Can sometimes remember things from the day before	Can sometimes remember events from earlier that day	Hardly ever remembers recent events
Long-term memory *Seems to talk most about memories from_____ period in life*	Remembers things well from middle age	Remembers things well from young adulthood	Remembers things from childhood, or little memory of past	Hardly ever seems to remember the past
Goal direction	Can remember the goal of most activities and complete steps to achieve goal	Can remember the goals of familiar activities and with help can complete steps to achieve goal	Can sometimes remember the goal of familiar activities, and can complete simple steps	Does not seem to remember or understand most familiar activities
Attention	Can sometimes concentrate for 30–60 minutes	Can sometimes concentrate for 15–30 minutes	Can sometimes concentrate for up to 15 minutes	Can sometimes concentrate for up to 5 minutes

	Typical dementia stage (rough guide, and people can have thinking abilities across different stages)			
	Mild dementia	Mild to moderate dementia	Moderate to severe dementia	Severe dementia
Decision making	Can choose from multiple options that are named but not shown	Can choose from multiple options that are shown	Can choose from two options that are shown	Does not usually make choices when offered
Communicating	Speaks using sentences, though may have difficulty finding the right words	Speaks using short phrases	Communicates using single words or through body language	Communicates through body language only
Understanding	Can follow a conversation of several sentences in a row	Can follow a conversation of one sentence at a time	Can follow a conversation using simple phrases and body language	Can understand single words (e.g. their name) and body language
Coordination abilities	Has good hand–eye coordination and can manipulate objects in complex sequences (e.g. tying a shoe lace)	Has good hand–eye coordination and can manipulate objects in complex sequences	Has reasonable hand–eye coordination and can manipulate objects in simple sequences	Has difficulty controlling hands and manipulating objects

Case study

Brian

Brian has moderate to severe fronto-temporal dementia. He lives in a nursing home.

1. Places of significance

Brian was born in the regional city of Orange, in central New South Wales, Australia, a well-known farming and agricultural region. He has lived there all his life.

2. People of significance

Brian never married. His nephews, Gary and Daniel, are involved in his care but don't report a close relationship with their uncle. Their father, Brian's brother, would have expected them to help look after Brian and they see it as their responsibility to be involved in his care. Brian has always been close to John, who was a school friend and then later his business partner.

3. Activities of significance

Brian's father was a butcher, so he apprenticed as a butcher, but later changed his mind and started working as a mechanic fixing farm machinery. He went on to start a farm machinery business with John. Brian does not currently undertake any activities.

4. Events of significance

Gary says that his uncle didn't talk much about his experiences in the Vietnam War, but he thought that this has probably affected him greatly. His uncle was a disciplinarian, placing value on respect and hard work.

5. Personal recreation preference

Gary said that his uncle was very close to John, who visits him weekly in the nursing home, but otherwise was a loner and didn't like being with people. He has never been close to his brothers and sisters and the rest of the family.

6. What is missing?

Gary rather vaguely says that Brian is missing everything that is important in his life now, although he's not sure if Brian really notices missing those things.

Here is the table for Brian. His short-term memory is relatively good compared to his other abilities, but he seems to have difficulty with attention and decision making.

| | Typical dementia stage (rough guide, and people can have thinking abilities across different stages) | | | |
	Mild dementia	Mild to moderate dementia	Moderate to severe dementia	Severe dementia
Short-term memory	Can sometimes remember things from the week before or better	Can sometimes remember things from the day before	Can sometimes remember events from earlier that day	Hardly ever remembers recent events
Long-term memory *Seems to talk most about memories from_____ period in life*	Remembers things well from middle age	Remembers things well from young adulthood	Remembers things from childhood, or little memory of past	Hardly ever seems to remember the past
			doesn't talk much, hard to answer	
Goal direction	Can remember the goal of most activities and complete steps to achieve goal	Can remember the goals of familiar activities and with help can complete steps to achieve goal	Can sometimes remember the goal of familiar activities, and can complete simple steps	Does not seem to remember or understand most familiar activities
Attention	Can sometimes concentrate for 30–60 minutes	Can sometimes concentrate for 15–30 minutes	Can sometimes concentrate for up to 15 minutes	Can sometimes concentrate for up to 5 minutes

| | Typical dementia stage (rough guide, and people can have thinking abilities across different stages) | | | |
	Mild dementia	Mild to moderate dementia	Moderate to severe dementia	Severe dementia
Decision making	Can choose from multiple options that are named but not shown	Can choose from multiple options that are shown	Can choose from two options that are shown	Does not usually make choices when offered
Communicating	Speaks using sentences, though may have difficulty finding the right words	Speaks using short phrases	Communicates using single words or through body language	Communicates through body language only
Understanding	Can follow a conversation of several sentences in a row	Can follow a conversation of one sentence at a time	Can follow a conversation using simple phrases and body language	Can understand single words (e.g. their name) and body language
Coordination abilities	Has good hand–eye coordination and can manipulate objects in complex sequences (e.g. tying a shoe lace)	Has good hand–eye coordination and can manipulate objects in complex sequences	Has reasonable hand–eye coordination and can manipulate objects in simple sequences	Has difficulty controlling hands and manipulating objects

3

SELECTING AND MODIFYING ACTIVITIES

As those of us who buy birthday or Christmas presents can attest, you can know someone quite well and still find it difficult to give them something they will like. And even if you think of something, it has to fit within your budget and be available for purchase. Similarly, even when you know a person with dementia well and understand their life history, it can be difficult to think of an activity that they may like to do. Any activity has to also be within the mental and physical capabilities of the person with dementia and meet logistical restrictions such as cost and transport.

BRAINSTORM POSSIBLE ACTIVITIES OR ACTIVITY THEMES

When you have collected the necessary information, you then need to brainstorm possible activities. When brainstorming, additionally take into account the reasons that you want to do activities with the person with dementia. If the main reason is so that the carer can spend quality time with the person with dementia, the list of activities may be very social. If the main reason is to try to get them exercising their brain, then cognitively stimulating activities may dominate the list. If the main reason is to help the person with dementia pass the time, then you may need a wider range of activities. If you are trying activities as a way of helping improve the behaviour of the person with dementia, then it may be helpful to try to understand why the person is behaving the way they do. While the activity may not directly address the causes or triggers for the behaviour, this understanding may help you to formulate the activities.

I like brainstorming by scribbling down as many ideas as possible relating to each aspect of the person's life history. After creating the list I can cancel out ones that are not feasible or are more difficult. I try not to immediately cancel out an idea because of logistical reasons, or because it is too 'hard' for the person with dementia, because these may be overcome with modifications to the activity or with more brainstorming.

I often find it helpful to think up ideas when working with someone else who knows the person with dementia, such as a family member or a professional carer. The nature of our relationship with the person with dementia often affects our ideas for activities. The activities a husband thinks of doing with his wife are sometimes different to those that a daughter would think of doing with her mother. A professional carer would develop different ideas for activities for that person, too.

Developing ideas for activities is a skill and becomes easier with practice. Some people seem to be able to come up with activities more intuitively and others have to work harder to develop their ideas. Some people with dementia are easier to think of activities for than others, too.

Case study

JOY

Bernie finds that Joy follows him around the house all the time. She doesn't start any activities of her own; he is concerned that she spends all her time watching him do things, and sometimes he finds her constant company and chatter tiring. Bernie would like to find some things they can do together and even some that she can do independently.

Bernie writes the following list of potential activities for Joy. Since Joy's cognitive ability is relatively preserved, his list contains many usual activities that are meaningful to her. He may have to modify these activities or provide extra support for Joy so that they are achievable.

Activities relating to places of significance:
- *Reminisce about or talk about Europe or France*

Activities relating to people of significance: —

Activities of significance (including present activities):
- *Listen to music*
- *Watch footage of movies and adverts Joy was in*
- *Read fashion magazines*

Activities relating to events of significance:
- *Go back to church where we got married*

Activities that may address things that are missing in her life:
- *Do something social (maybe invite Martin and Meredith for dinner?)*
- *Go shopping and for lunch (I could take her, but not sure how this would work)*

ANTONIO

Maria is worried that Antonio spends a lot of the time sitting around doing nothing. Sometimes he disappears into his shed; however, she thinks he doesn't do much in the shed either. Antonio used to go to the café and have coffee with other retired Italian gentlemen, but when his memory started to deteriorate he stopped going. She says that he is still capable of going on his usual evening walk by himself, but he doesn't go any more. When she suggests that he go for a walk, he says he would rather stay home with her.

Maria says that Antonio was always such a busy man, working on their business or helping with the soccer club or other Italian community events. Maria says that she has a lot of work to do around the house and Antonio is always sleeping while she cleans and cooks. Maria spends a lot of time helping her daughters by sometimes transporting their children to activities, cooking and doing laundry and sewing. Maria is not sure what to do with Antonio when she is out of the house, and he often doesn't want to come with her when she goes out. Antonio had reasonable conversational English but this has deteriorated with his dementia. This means that his grandchildren find it difficult to communicate with him because even though they have been taught Italian, they are not fluent or confident in the language.

Maria and her daughter Sofia brainstorm some activities that they can do with Antonio. Many of these are cognitively stimulating, because Maria is particularly concerned about Antonio's declining memory and thinking abilities. Their brainstormed list looks like this:

Activities relating to places of significance:

- *Something to do with Italian culture/language*
- *Maybe help Sofia's son Tony with Italian homework?*
- *Or go to Italian club for lunch more regularly, though he didn't like doing that in the past*

Activities relating to people of significance: —

Activities of significance (including present activities):

- *Something to do with Brunswick Juventus*
- *Look at old photo albums of team, or newspaper clippings*
- *Talk about old players*
- *Go to watch soccer game — or watch on television*
- *Get Antonio to talk to Tony about Brunswick Juventus*
- *Something relating to convenience-store business*
- *Grocery catalogues — read them and comment on prices? Not sure if this will be meaningful?*
- *Or grocery catalogues, black out prices and ask him to guess?*
- *Or simple ledger and get him to add up maths? Maybe too hard?*
- *Go shopping with Maria and comment on the business or shop layout?*
- *Do 'inventory' of items in home pantry? Will probably need help with this as pantry is a bit of a mess*
- *Go for walks with different family members*

Activities relating to events of significance: —

Activities relating to things missing in his life: —

RUTH

Ruth is fairly independent in self-care. However since moving into the nursing home she constantly demands the attention of the staff. She wants to be with staff all the time and is constantly seeking emotional and physical reassurance. She talks about being worried that something is wrong, though when questioned cannot be specific about what this is. Ruth sometimes goes into the rooms of the other residents and takes their belongings. She also often hovers around the staff office and work areas, trying to get into those spaces. She also spends a lot of time wandering around at night.

Ruth's daughters, Julie and Hannah, visit weekly. When they visit, Ruth is happy and affectionate. She likes going for a walk to the onsite café for a sweet treat. She usually gets upset when they leave. However, when they reassure her that they need to go to work or collect their children and will be back soon, she will let them go, with a few tears. Ruth also likes going for walks with Julie and Hannah around the small garden in the unit. Julie and Hannah notice that Ruth does not particularly like talking about the past; both suspect that she cannot remember much about her life. They have the same conversation each time when Ruth asks why her other daughter, Jane, hasn't been to see her for a while, and Ruth is always surprised to learn that Jane lives in England and isn't planning to come back. Ruth always then says: 'Jane won't like the cold, she will be back soon, you'll see.'

Nursing-home staff try to occupy Ruth so that she is not so disruptive to the other residents. They give her socks and handkerchiefs to fold and sort as an activity.

However she only does these tasks with company, and only for a few minutes before getting up and wanting to do something else. Ruth refuses to join in group activities such as flower arranging or craft, and does not like looking at photo albums or watching television. Ruth does, however, like arranging the baby dolls in their cot in the lounge room, but she will not let any of the other residents touch them or hold them. Ruth's behaviour has caused some conflict with other residents, who are bothered by her constant hovering and interfering with their belongings, and dominance of the dolls.

The unit nurses discuss Ruth's unsettled behaviour with Julie and Hannah and ask if they could bring in some things that Ruth liked doing at home, which might occupy her. Julie and Hannah talk about things that Ruth might still do, and they struggle to think of much. They can think of many outings or activities that Ruth would like to do with them, but not much that she could do by herself. Their list looks like this:

Activities relating to places of significance: —

Activities relating to people of significance:
- *Visits from Julie and Hannah, maybe the grandchildren can visit more regularly*
- *Maybe go to Julie's or Hannah's for lunch?*

Activities of significance (including present activities):
- *Knitting*
- *Reading (romance novels)*

Activities relating to events of significance: —

Activities relating to things missing in her life: —

Note: If you are the family carer of a person who lives in a nursing home, you may also have difficulty thinking of activities that the person with dementia can do alone. This is because people with dementia usually need support to complete activities successfully. It may be unrealistic to expect people to do activities alone. Talk to the facility staff about whether they have a little time each day to do an individualized activity with the person with dementia, or at least start and supervise an activity for them. Do activities with your loved one yourself so that facility staff can observe the benefits of the activity for your loved one. Request politely that the time be found. There may be volunteers who visit the facility who may be able to do the activity with the person with dementia. Work with the facility staff to find activities for the person with dementia that will work within the time restrictions and capabilities of facility staff. Educate the facility about what the person with dementia enjoys and the need for activities for the person. Do this with respect and understanding and appreciation of the care the facility provides for your loved one.

BRIAN

Brian's behaviour in the nursing home is unpredictable. Sometimes he is extremely apathetic. He seems completely switched off from the world, sitting still for hours with his head hung low, eyes closed. When he is this way it is difficult to get his attention or get him to participate in a conversation or move from his seat. Other times, he becomes suddenly enraged and it is not always clear why. He lashes out by yelling and being physically threatening to both the nursing-home staff and his nephews when they come to visit. Staff report that Brian seems to be happiest when his friend John visits, though he can be even more moody and uncooperative afterwards.

Brian's nephews Gary and Daniel find visits very challenging and yet feel a sense of obligation to keep on visiting him. 'Why go and see the old bugger if he just yells and cusses us?' says Daniel. 'He's better off without us visiting, and better for us too.' Brian often doesn't seem to recognize his nephews or their wives. They find it difficult to chat with him and have very short visits. Gary and Daniel decide to try to improve the quality of their visits with Brian. They have seen other families looking at photographs and bringing gifts made by their grandchildren.

Gary and Daniel struggle to think up anything they can do with Brian given his level of cognitive impairment. June, Gary's wife, suggests bringing a photo album, though Gary is doubtful they will get any sense out of Brian about the photos; he has never been a sentimental man. June also suggests that they take Brian on an outing, but Gary says that this is too difficult and that Brian will probably not care about going out anyway. Not surprisingly, their brainstormed list is short:

Activities relating to places of significance: —

Activities relating to people of significance:
- *Look at old photo albums?*

Activities of significance (including present activities):
- Go for a walk?

Activities relating to events of significance: —

Activities relating to things missing in his life: —

Note: You may find that, like Brian's family, you find it hard initially to brainstorm many ideas for activities. If this is the case, don't worry! Reading through this book may give you some inspiration. If you have one idea, then that is a start. I almost always find that when I'm doing an activity with a person with dementia, I find out more about things they seem to be interested in, or are able to do, and get other ideas. You'll read more about this in the section on trialling activities. People with moderate to severe dementia might not need a variety of different activities; between one and three that they enjoy may be enough, and too many activities could be confusing for them.

REFINE YOUR BRAINSTORMED LIST OF ACTIVITIES

I wouldn't expect a two-year-old to complete a 30-piece jigsaw puzzle herself.

I wouldn't expect a second-year medical student to conduct an appendectomy himself.

I wouldn't expect a person with moderate dementia to cook a meal themselves.

But all these people can meaningfully participate in and contribute to the task in some way. The two-year-old might turn the jigsaw pieces so they all face up, and help match some of the pieces and physically connect the pieces together. The medical student could observe the procedure and help conduct and record the patient observations. The person with dementia can chop the vegetables, stir the pot, taste and comment on the levels of seasoning, and help serve the meal.

The first step in modifying an activity is to work out the different steps in the activity. Then for each step, figure out what the person can do independently, what they may have difficulty with and what you don't think they can manage at all. The first time you do this 'task analysis' it is easier to write down the steps. Next to each step, write your guess about whether the person with dementia can do the step, or how you can modify the step to make it easier for them. As you become familiar with this process, you can stop writing down the task analysis. However, if you are a professional carer working in a team, it may be useful to continue to write down the information to share with colleagues.

Case study

ANTONIO

Maria and Sofia write down a task analysis for taking an inventory of their home pantry. They are surprised at how many steps this relatively 'simple' job has. They also identify steps where Antonio would have difficulty.

1. **Create a table on a piece of paper in which to write the inventory.** *He may not know how to lay out the table, I'm not sure he will remember what needs to happen on an inventory list. Antonio probably needs verbal instructions to help with this step.*

2. **Get some cardboard boxes.** *He probably won't think of organizing himself this way, he would just take everything out and put it on the table, and when he runs out of space he'll put things on the kitchen benches and on the floor and it would be a*

big mess. Antonio probably needs regular verbal instructions to help with this step.

3. **Take out each item from the pantry and check the condition of the packaging. If it is damaged, throw it away. If the condition looks fine, check the use-by date. If it is expired, throw it away.** *If it is within the date, store in cardboard box. I think he would know how to do this, as long as we write down the current date somewhere he can see it. We'd also have to put the bin out somewhere close by. Antonio probably needs supervision to help with this step.*

4. **Place each item by category into the cardboard boxes. If there is no cardboard box that seems appropriate, decide where to put it.** *I think he may not do this correctly, but I suppose it doesn't matter. If we labelled each cardboard box with a category of items from the pantry (e.g. baking supplies, pasta) this might help him. Antonio probably needs supervision to help with this step.*

5. **When all items have been removed from the pantry, wipe down the shelves with a cleaning product, then with water.** *He should be able to do this if we suggest it. Antonio probably needs supervision to help with this step.*

6. **Write down the name of each item, and count the number of each. Transfer each item from one box to another in order to keep track of what has been written down and counted.** *He could do all the writing, but we have a big pantry, I think there would be too many items for him to inventory. Just doing a few would be enough. Antonio probably needs supervision to start to help with this step.*

7. **Decide where each group of items will be stored in the pantry based on size and frequency of use.** *He wouldn't know the best places for things to go, because he doesn't cook. He also may not remember where they used to go. I think he might have trouble making a decision, even if it doesn't matter what he decides. And he might not remember where he had decided things should go. Antonio probably needs regular verbal instructions to help with this step, though it might just be too hard for him.*

8. **Return items to pantry, arranging them so that the labels face the front and they are stacked neatly.** *I think he would be able to do this easily if told where to put them. Antonio probably needs supervision to help with this step.*

9. **Take the rubbish out and put away the empty cardboard boxes.** *I think he would be able to do this easily if told where to put them. Antonio probably needs supervision to help with this step.*

After conducting the task analysis, Maria and Sofia decide it is probably too big a task for Antonio to conduct an inventory of the pantry, even with help. They decide to divide the activity into two: cleaning out the pantry with the supervision and instructions provided by Maria, and inventorying some items that Maria will preselect (just Step 6 from the list above). We will hear how Antonio and Maria go with these activities later.

ONGOING MODIFICATION OF ACTIVITIES

Planning a modification of an activity is the first part of modification. The second part is adapting the activity 'on the fly' during the activity with the person with dementia. When we do the task analysis, we guess what the person with dementia is able to do, but our guesses will probably not all be right. When this happens, we will have to improvise and modify the activity by providing more support or making the step simpler. We might also find that we've made the activity too easy or too short and the person with dementia wants to continue. In this case, we will also have to improvise and repeat the activity with a variation, or quickly think up a whole new activity to do!

Once a person with dementia has done an activity several times he will often 'learn' it, even if he doesn't remember doing it before. When this happens, you will need to vary the activity or modify it to make it more challenging.

HOW MUCH SUPPORT TO GIVE WITH AN ACTIVITY

There are two different schools of thought as to how much support to give a person with dementia when doing an activity with them. Some experts suggest giving the minimal amount of support possible so as to empower the person and help them maintain their independence. Other experts suggest that it is good communication practice to always model an activity for a person with dementia, and that this gives good results in helping the person understand and do the activity.

I think that both approaches have their merits and you could choose either approach. If you are doing the activity because you want to mentally stimulate and challenge the person with dementia, or the activity is a way of them practising skills to help them maintain their independence, then give as little support as necessary. However, if you're doing the activity for enjoyment, then you may want to maximize the chance of them starting the activity by making it very clear what the activity is through demonstration. I tend to take the first approach of maximizing independence for people with mild dementia, and the approach of maximizing success for people with moderate to severe dementia.

The list below gives information about the different amount of help or support that a person with dementia may need on a task, going from least help to most help.

1. Independent. No help required; person with dementia can do the whole step themselves including initiating it.

2. Supervision. The person with dementia may need supervision for initiation, safety, comfort and if they run into an unexpected difficulty.

3. Occasional verbal prompt. The person with dementia might need help staying on task or to make decisions with the help of verbal instructions such as 'What do you need to do now?' or 'The next step is ...'

4. Regular verbal instructions. The person with dementia needs ongoing verbal instructions on how to do the task.

5. Verbal instructions and gestures. The person with dementia cannot follow verbal instructions alone and requires physical explanation as well. For instance, you might need to point to the items they

need, or mimic the motions (without using the objects) they should be doing, e.g. stirring.

6. Copying. The person with dementia needs to watch another person demonstrate the step before undertaking it; e.g. you might say: 'Watch me; now it's your turn.'

7. Physical help. The person with dementia may need physical help to complete the step; e.g. you might need to guide their hand to pick up the wooden spoon and stir the bowl with your hand over theirs.

TRIALLING ACTIVITIES

You don't know how interested the person with dementia is going to be in the activities that you've brainstormed. He or she may love it, dislike it or be uninterested. You can try to judge interest simply by asking the person whether they think they'd like the activity, but often we've found that people with dementia will refuse to go out, or to try something new, but when cajoled into doing it they really enjoy it.

So the best way to judge interest is to try an activity with them. It is usually clear from the first few minutes of an activity (once you're got the person doing it) whether they are engaged and enjoying it or not. Always have a 'back-up' activity if possible to fall back on in case they dislike the activity. This may be a conversation topic that they like or even a snack or meal to engage their attention.

Case study

ANTONIO

Maria gives Antonio the inventory activity to do. She gets out of the pantry multiple packets of pasta and cans of beans. She also creates an inventory list that is a similar, simplified version of the one they used in their convenience store. She places the food products on the dining table with the objects to the right of where Antonio usually sits, and the list in front of his usual chair. This conversation occurred in Italian.

Maria: 'Antonio, can you help me with this job, please?'

Antonio: 'What do you want me to do?'

Maria: 'I need to inventory this stock.'

Antonio: 'There isn't much there.'

Maria: 'I know. Would you mind please helping me write the names and numbers down on this inventory sheet?'

Antonio walks over.

Maria: (patting the seat) 'Sit down here.'

Antonio: 'What do you want me to do?'

Maria: 'Write down the names of each product on this list. What is the name of that packet in front of you?'

Antonio: 'Heinz tomato sauce.'

Maria: (placing the pen in Antonio's hand and then pointing) 'Write here ... Heinz tomato sauce.

Put all the ones you've written down on this side. You do one.'

Antonio takes a packet, reads the name and writes it down. Maria watches while he adds several items to the list.

Maria: 'That's it. Good. Okay, I will be cooking in the kitchen.'

When Maria returns from the kitchen in 20 minutes, she finds Antonio still sitting at the kitchen table. He is looking confused and has his head in his hands. He has written about ten products down on the sheet; several are repeated and then crossed out. He keeps picking up a product, looking at the name, looking at the list and then putting it down again.

Maria: 'Hello, my darling.'

Antonio: 'I can't do it.'

Maria: 'What can't you do?'

Antonio: 'I don't know.'

Maria: 'Don't worry about it, darling.' (takes his hand) 'Come into the lounge and we'll watch television together.'

The next week, Maria tries the same activity again, but this time she sets it up in the kitchen so that she can help Antonio if he has any difficulty. She makes sure she places products that have been written down to the side, and also reminds him what he is doing. This time he completes it successfully and she thanks him for his help.

The next day, Maria gives Antonio the inventory list, to which she has added prices. She also has some sticky labels. Together, they label the products with hand-written labels. Antonio reads each product off the list, Maria selects it from the table, Antonio then writes the label and sticks it onto the product.

The above example shows the importance of trialling the whole activity with the person with dementia. Antonio seemed happy and able to do the activity, so Maria left him unsupervised. She did not anticipate that he would get confused and forget which items he had already inventoried. This example shows how when people with dementia are not supported to ensure that the activity is achievable they can become distressed at their apparent failure.

Even though the activity wasn't successful for Antonio the first time, Maria thought that with modification the activity might still work and tried it again with success. Maria felt it was somehow more normal to both be working at the kitchen table and that they could 'chat' about their tasks as they had previously done in their business. Maria also modified and extended the inventory activity to make it a price labelling activity.

It is possible that after Antonio had done the inventory activity a few times he may have been able to complete it without Maria being present; she could have given less and less support to see if he could learn to do the activity unsupervised. Labels on the table in front of each group of items, stating 'not inventoried items' and 'inventoried items', may have helped in reducing the supervision needed.

Case study

RUTH

Hannah and Julie take Ruth's knitting bag with a half-completed jumper to the nursing home, along with a few romance novels that she used to enjoy. Ruth takes the knitting out of the basket, but after looking at it for a while puts it away and doesn't do any knitting at all. She looks at the novels and then puts them down without opening them. Her behaviour continues as before. The unit nurse takes out the knitting on another occasion and tries to encourage her to knit, but Ruth refuses. The staff thought that Ruth could no longer knit.

A week later, an activity officer, Kata, spends some one-on-one time with Ruth. Kata brings a book of knitting patterns for babies. She thinks that, given Ruth's interest in the baby dolls, she might enjoy looking at the pictures of the cute babies. Kata also wants to see how interested Ruth may be in the topic of knitting.

To introduce the activity Kata tells Ruth that her brother is having a baby and asks for her help in choosing a pattern to knit. Ruth turns the pages of the book and comments on the patterns, explaining which patterns are easy and which more difficult. She also recommends knitting a cardigan as it is easier to put on, and comments that the mother would appreciate the cardigan but the baby wouldn't! She then offers to knit a toy from the book for the baby.

During the afternoon craft activity, having built a rapport with Ruth earlier, Kata tries to persuade Ruth to sit with the other residents and participate, but she again refuses.

The next week Kata brings a ball of wool and knitting needles of the right size for the wool. She sits next to Ruth at the table where she is having morning tea and puts the wool and needles on the table. She is about to start knitting to see if she can persuade Ruth to talk about knitting, or reminisce about knitting more, when Ruth says, 'So, you want to learn to knit?' She then proceeds to cast on and gives Kata a lesson on how to knit and purl, and talks about garter stitch, stocking stitch and ribbing. Ruth's hands seem to work on auto pilot. She gets confused with some of her explanations, makes some mistakes in her own knitting, but this is not important. She goes on to explain how to measure for a jumper and figure out how many stitches to cast on — while the explanation doesn't fully make sense it is clear what she is explaining. Kata doesn't have to talk much or do much throughout the whole interaction, except to try to knit a few times, after which Ruth takes over to 'show' her again. It is as if Kata has switched on a knitting teaching program in Ruth's behavioural vocabulary. The other care staff are amazed at Ruth's knitting and also her animation and confidence in teaching Kata.

Kata tries to leave the knitting with Ruth but she refuses. She tells Kata she isn't doing it for her, and she needs to go and practise. She agrees to show Kata some more knitting the next time she comes to visit.

The next week, Kata spends one-on-one time with Ruth again. She asks Ruth to demonstrate ribbing. While Ruth knits and explains she also talks about her husband

and children and the items she knitted for them (socks for her husband's very big feet). During the afternoon cooking activity Kata persuades Ruth to sit with the group, however after a few minutes she gets up and walks away. Ruth is more easily persuaded to sit with the group during their craft activity, however again she does not stay long. They never manage to persuade Ruth to join in with group activities.

Kata phones Julie. She suggests that they try to facilitate Ruth knitting squares to make a blanket. Julie agrees to buy yarn and needles. Julie also knits a sample square, writes out a pattern for the square and titles it 'Squares for Julie's blanket'. She also casts on the first square for Ruth. Julie then takes the materials to show Ruth. She asks Ruth if she would help her knit a blanket and Ruth agrees. She gives the cast-on square to Ruth and starts another square herself.

Later that afternoon, staff find Ruth still knitting the square. The next day, they bring her the knitting and ask her to continue knitting the blanket for Julie. By the next day, the square has become a rectangle and Ruth keeps knitting. She needs help a few times when she loses a needle or drops a stitch, but she sits for 10 to 15 minutes knitting as long as a staff member is there keeping her company before carefully putting away her work in the bag. She responds best to Kata but will also knit when invited by other staff. When Julie visits she finishes off the rectangle and starts Ruth on another square. This continues until they have enough rectangles and squares, and Julie sews them up into a blanket which is placed on Ruth's bed. They then start another blanket. The main

problem for staff is finding where Ruth has put the
knitting bag each time.

The above example shows the importance of modifying activities
before trialling them. The activity needs to be presented in a
way which is meaningful and tailored so that it is achievable.
Ruth had no interest in completing the half-knitted jumper that
she may not have recognized as her own, and the pattern may
have been too complex for her to follow. Kata started off with a
discussion about knitting and discovered that Ruth still showed
an interest in the activity. Ruth needed someone to initiate
knitting, and also to keep her on track with the activity. Kata was
sensitive and skilled in providing this. Ruth had both motor and
procedural memory for plain knitting that surpassed the staff's
expectations. The rationale of knitting a blanket for Julie was
sufficient to at least get her started each time, after which the
motor memory and enjoyment of the process probably kept her
knitting for some time.

4

PRESENTING AND SCHEDULING ACTIVITIES

You cannot learn to ski by reading a book (or even a hundred books) about skiing. The first time you go on a ski slope you almost certainly will fall down. Similarly, reading this book will not instantly make you an expert at presenting activities for a person with dementia. However, I hope that after reading this chapter you will be able to present an activity successfully. There will be occasions when interactions will not work as well as you imagined they would, and you will learn from these experiences even more than you learn from your successes.

TALK LESS, WATCH MORE!

When communicating with people with dementia remember to talk less and watch more! This principle works well in any situation where communication is difficult, such as where there is a lot of noise and conversation can't be heard well, when talking with very young children or even when trying to have a conversation with a teenager.

Watch the person with dementia more

Movement is the earliest form of communication we have. Seventy per cent of our communication is based on body language. We learn to rely on language in understanding others but sometimes we over-rely on it, focusing too much on the words and forgetting about body language. For instance, the wife of an unfaithful husband might have realized something was wrong earlier if she had been more aware of how his body language and tone reflected his feelings towards her, rather than just relying on his words.

Language enhances our ability to communicate information about the past and in the future; it lets us converse about more complex and metaphysical topics. Once we've developed physical speech, vocabulary and grammar between the ages of one and five, we assume that language is the key to communication. Language is a way of encoding the world, and many of our memories of the world are coded in words. Talking is the part of communication that requires the most conscious effort. Sometimes we struggle to find the right words to say when hearing bad news, when we could use our face and a hug or touch to convey our reaction.

There are many situations where ideas and feelings are conveyed without words. Mime artists and dancers convey complex stories through body language. People with dementia convey a great deal of information through their face and body, how they hold themselves and how they move. We need to watch and read this information, since people with dementia often have difficulty using words.

Tone and pitch are also important parts of communication. Babies communicate their moods and needs using a range of sounds such as cries, gurgles and coos. Animals communicate in their social groups and hierarchies through body language and tone and pitch. We can tell if a dog is scared or is being aggressive or friendly through the tone of its bark or whine. When we listen to the person with dementia talk, listen not just to decipher the meaning of the words, but also for the feelings conveyed through tone.

Watch your own mood more

Our moods affect how we behave, and awareness of our own moods helps minimize the chance of inadvertently putting out negative vibes. You may have had a poor night's sleep and be slightly impatient because of this. Perhaps you have a headache or toothache that is making you grumpy or irritable. You could be feeling sad or angry because of some personal event in your life. However, the person with dementia does not know why you are behaving impatiently, irritably or angrily. They may think your mood reflects your attitude towards them or their behaviour in some way.

Family carers often feel guilt, loss, sadness and even anger towards a person with dementia because of their condition and the stressors of the caregiving role. Professional carers may feel irritated, annoyed or frustrated towards the person with dementia because they see them as uncooperative, rude or ungrateful. These feelings are all understandable given the situation. However, negative feelings get in the way of good interactions with the person with dementia. The person with dementia will pick up on the emotion, even if they don't realize the reason for it, and react to that emotion.

Another reason to be aware of and manage our own moods is that people with dementia mirror the emotions of those around them. We all do this to some extent, but this emotional contagion is much more pronounced in people with mild dementia than those without dementia. We don't know exactly why this happens, but scientists think it could be because the person with dementia is trying to fit in socially, and since they are less able to understand the meaning of the words being spoken they compensate by responding to the emotions.

In order to manage my mood, I like to take in a deep breath and hold it, then exhale and relax my body before I enter a room or start an interaction or conversation with a person with dementia. I also find it helpful to stay present in the moment with the person I'm interacting with. If I know I'm in a mood I find difficult to ignore, then I try to choose an activity that is easier for me to present or that is dependent on objects the person with dementia looks at and manipulates, and is less dependent on my interaction with the person with dementia.

Throughout the encounter with the person with dementia, we also need to keep up our awareness of our moods. I find some people with dementia more difficult to be with than others, particularly those with very unpredictable behaviours or strong negative moods. I sometimes find myself getting bothered by repetitive yelling or constant demands for attention. In these cases I remind myself to be calm and that the person is not behaving that way to annoy me, but rather is most probably expressing a need for help, or attention, or company, or reassurance or some physical discomfort. I try to connect with the person in order to try to change their behaviour.

I sometimes feel frustrated or disappointed when an activity does not go as planned and I am unable to connect with someone or they do not seem to want my company or say negative things about me. However, I try not to take these occurrences as personal rejections or as a failure on my part. Rather, I remind myself that things cannot always go to plan and try to use the situation as a learning experience. I try to identify where things did not work so well and plan a new approach the next time.

I find it useful to debrief and talk about an interaction that has brought up an emotional reaction within me, usually with a colleague. If you are a family carer, try to find a relative or friend who will understand and debrief. Debriefing helps us process and deal with negative feelings, and helps us prepare for next time.

Watch your own behaviour more

We are often careful about choosing our words but sometimes we realize that we've said the wrong thing and want to take the words back. Occasionally we realize that even though the words were fine, our tone was not appropriate and we apologize: 'Sorry I yelled at you, I was a bit stressed about getting the job done on time.' However, we rarely reflect on our body language and what message it is sending. I have never heard anyone say, 'Sorry I didn't give you eye contact, but I really didn't want to hear about your bowels again,' or 'Sorry my face looked so dour and stern, I didn't know how to react to your news.'

People with dementia often forget the words you have said to them and sometimes cannot follow the meanings of the sentences. However, they can read your body language and tone as these are more basic forms of communication. We need to be much more aware of our bodies, faces and gestures and consciously use them to communicate in a relaxed and positive way with people with dementia.

If the person with dementia is sitting down, do not stand over them; this can sometimes seem threatening or suggest that you may not stay long. Ask her permission to sit next to her, and pull up a chair. If there is nowhere to sit I often kneel beside the person. I prefer to sit beside or at a right angle to the person with dementia rather than directly opposite, which can sometimes feel too intimate or intense. It is also easier to look at something together if we are sitting alongside each other.

I described earlier the way people with dementia subconsciously mirror the emotions of those around them, possibly in an effort to fit in socially. We can use this strategy consciously to connect better with the person with dementia by mirroring the speed and intensity of the person with dementia. Match your speed to the speed of the person with dementia. The speed at which they move and talk reflects the pace at which they are thinking, which is also the pace at which they can absorb and process information. This means that we need to slow down when interacting with most people with dementia — sometimes we need to *slow right down*.

It's also important to match your intensity of pitch and movement to the intensity and mood of the person with dementia. When someone else is displaying the same mood that we are, or seems to be in emotional synchrony with us, we feel more rapport with and more positively towards that person. We find it easier to relate to them and feel more involved and compatible with people with whom we are sharing the same mood. This occurs irrespective of whether the shared mood is negative or positive. If the person with dementia is moving with a great deal of positive energy, I try to be high energy and happy too. If the person with dementia seems to have low energy and mood, I try to be calm, present and subdued, though not negative in my mood. It can be grating when we are feeling sad or low to interact with someone who is obnoxiously happy.

Obviously we do not mirror the person with dementia's mood when they are displaying an intensely negative mood, such as anger, distress or extreme sadness. In that case, always model the mood you wish them to be in, i.e. calm and relaxed.

Talk less

Only about 10 per cent of communication is based on the words we use. But these words can be very useful! When communication is difficult we tend to talk more. If the person we are talking to doesn't understand what we're saying then we often say it again. Then we may rephrase it and elaborate, and sometimes in this elaboration we talk both faster and louder. And then we say it again ... and again! This strategy may work sometimes but it does not work for people with dementia.

Talk less when communicating with people with dementia. Choose your words carefully and use short sentences and simple phrases. Think before you speak, and make every word count (like a tweet!).

WHAT TO TALK ABOUT WITH PEOPLE WITH DEMENTIA

I have had many interesting and enjoyable conversations with people with dementia. However, many people struggle to have a conversation with a person with dementia. Many of our conversations with friends and family start with one person asking a question to which the person responds by reporting their news and there is some discussion around this. The other person then reciprocates by asking a question of the first person which generates more discussion. Both people get to talk about themselves or their lives or interests. This usually happens before the conversation progresses onto other topics.

Here is the pattern:

Person 1: Question?

Person 2: Answer.

Person 1: Response to answer.

Person 2: Response to answer. Question?

Person 1: Answer.

Person 2: Response to answer.

Here is an example:

Betty: 'How was your holiday?'

Lucy: 'It was wonderful ... the weather was
           surprisingly good and Tasmania is really
           beautiful. Have you met my cousin
           Charley? We stayed with him for a week in
           Hobart and the birds come to his backyard
           every morning and he feeds them. I don't
           know if that is allowed, but anyway ...'

Betty: 'I've never been to Tasmania, I'd like to go
           sometime.'

Lucy: 'I recommend you go. It was a wonderful
           trip ... How about you? What have you been
           up to?'

Betty: 'Well, we have been busy with the garden.
           One of the big trees got a disease and we
           had to get it removed as it was in danger
           of falling. What an expensive exercise that
           was, and we had to get permission from the
           council too.'

Lucy: 'Our friend wanted to cut down a tree
           to improve his view and he had to get
           permission from the council too. He really
           had trouble getting permission. It's his

garden and his tree, why would he need permission? I don't remember how he got permission eventually, but the view at his place is great now.'

If we try to start a conversation following this usual pattern with a person with dementia it often does not succeed. People with dementia often cannot remember 'news' to report. They also often do not have the initiative to ask questions of the other person.

Case study

JOY

In the example below, Betty is talking to Joy, who has mild Alzheimer's dementia. Joy has trouble responding and Betty finds the lack of input from Joy difficult, so she starts just talking about herself and dominating the conversation.

Betty: 'How was your holiday?'

Joy: 'We have not gone anywhere for a long time. We have stayed home.'

Betty.   'You did go on holiday, you were going to Cairns, remember?'

Joy: 'We haven't been to Cairns for years, we haven't been anywhere for a long time.'

Betty: 'I thought you went last month to Cairns, and stayed by the beach and took a boat trip?'

Joy:	'No, I don't think so.'
Betty:	'We used to take our children to the beach every school holidays. We would stay on the beach in this little house, the same one very time, like a home away from home. The children would get very brown — we didn't use sunscreen like they do these days — and put sand all through the house.'
Joy:	'Um … yes.'
Betty:	'I have been very busy around the garden lately …' (talks about garden)

Here are some tips for being a successful conversation partner for people with dementia.

- Don't ask questions about recent events or questions on topics that require information from their short-term memory.
- Ask about broad topics in their past that they probably remember, but not about specific details of events.
- Ask about topics that you know they like talking about.
- If they bring up a topic, encourage them to talk more about it. Listen for little clues about topics towards which you can steer the conversation. For instance, in our next example with Betty and Joy (see p. 91), after Joy talked about Bernie buying her roses when they were courting, Betty could have asked about how Bernie and Joy met, or what their courtship was like, or whether Bernie was a romantic person.
- Ask their advice. Ask their opinion on both small

dilemmas and big problems. 'What should I cook for dinner tonight?' or 'Should I let my sixteen-year-old daughter go on a date with a boy?'

- Talk about things in the present — things you can see, hear, smell and taste — the scene in front of you, the sound of the birds, the smell of the flowers or the taste of the cake you're sharing.

- Don't correct the person with dementia or argue about facts. If the person with dementia is talking about his past and says he has no grandchildren when he actually has three, it would be critical and disempowering to tell him he is wrong or has remembered that fact incorrectly.

- Remember that the person has difficulty with memory and other aspects of thinking, but they are not stupid! Don't talk to them as if they are stupid.

- Don't try to use absolute logic to convince them of something — though sometimes logic works if consistent with their world view. For instance, I was told a story about a man with dementia who was trying to leave home because he was convinced he was going to be late to work to meet the delivery truck. He wouldn't believe his wife when she said that he no longer went to work. However, in keeping with his current world view, his wife told him the delivery truck driver had called, had explained they had broken down and were running late and would not arrive until the following morning. He consequently calmed down.

Case study

JOY

Here is an example of a conversation where Betty has taken a different approach to having a conversation with Joy. She does not rely on Joy's memory and creates opportunities for Joy to talk about topics she is interested in. She also does not expect that Joy will invite her to talk about herself. Many of the meaningful conversations of people with dementia are based on their established knowledge either of facts or their personal history. This is elaborated on further in the section on reminiscence.

Betty:	'Bernie told me that you've been on holidays to Cairns.'
Joy:	'We haven't been to Cairns for years, we haven't been anywhere for a long time.'
Betty:	'Tell me about what Cairns was like.'
Joy:	'Well, Bernie liked to go fishing when we went on holiday. He has always liked fishing. Sometimes I would go with him and sit in the boat, or sit on the beach with a book. It is nice sitting looking at the water. Do you know my husband Bernie?'
Betty:	'Yes I do.'
Joy:	'Well, you know that he is a tall man, he always says that I'm half the lady he is.' (laughs)
Betty:	(laughs) 'How did you and Bernie meet?'
Joy:	'We met on a train. We'd been catching the

same train into the city each day, and one morning it was raining and I had forgotten my umbrella, so Bernie walked me to my office. He was very handsome and tall, very tall. He walked me back to the train station that afternoon even though it wasn't raining. He walked me every day for a week, then asked me out to dinner.'

Here is another example of a conversation between Betty and Joy. Betty starts the conversation based on the weather, and asks Joy a general question not reliant on short-term memory.

Betty: 'It's a beautiful sunny day outside.'

Joy: 'Yes, it's nice to see the sunshine.'

Betty: 'The wisteria is just starting to bloom. That's my favourite flower. What is your favourite flower?'

Joy: 'Hmm ... I think it's roses. Yes. I like roses, with their many petals. Of course, the roses I like the best are the ones that Bernie used to buy me when we were courting.'

Betty: 'I'm going to tell him he has to buy you some more roses.'

Joy: 'No, I'm an old lady now, too old for courting.'

Betty: 'But not too old for roses!'

IT IS OKAY TO LIE TO A PERSON WITH DEMENTIA?

The ethics of lying are complex. My opinion is that perfect honesty is less important than respect, compassion and empathy. I take the utilitarian philosophical perspective that lying is acceptable when the resulting consequences maximize benefit or minimize harm, though it can be often very difficult to foresee what the consequence of a lie is going to be, and in those circumstances it is difficult to decide whether or not it is acceptable to lie.

I believe that persons with dementia should be protected from the outside world if they cannot cope with it. My pragmatic experience is that sometimes telling the person with dementia the truth does not help them and can actually distress them more. Telling the person with dementia a falsehood consistent with their beliefs may be better for their wellbeing. But withholding knowledge from the person with dementia takes away choices from them, and takes away their human right of freedom of information. So I try to foresee the consequences of the lie.

Take, for example, the issue of whether to remind a woman with dementia that her husband has passed away if she has forgotten this fact. If told, she will have to relive the experience of the grief of the initial loss of her husband and may be happier and better off continuing to believe her spouse is still alive. So in this case I would not usually remind the person that their spouse has passed away. However, if the person with dementia needs to make decisions about their life or estate, and needs to know that her husband has passed away as part of these decisions, then I would remind her about her husband's death.

There are some circumstances where, I feel, it is ethically acceptable to lie to a person with dementia, and in such cases you would need to balance protecting the feelings of the person with dementia with their right to know and any loss of freedom to make choices based on the information.

STATUS, CHOICE AND LETTING THE PERSON WITH DEMENTIA GIVE BACK

Social status refers to the rank or position of a person within a group, where a group could be just two people. Social status can be ascribed based on age, wealth, sex or ethnic group. Status can also be achieved through accumulation of knowledge or achievements. Within any group interaction, different people may have different levels of status dictated either through formal roles (e.g. the boss or the nominated leader, the group chair, the parent) or roles constrained by the situation (e.g. irate customer in relation to customer service officer, bank manager in relation to loan applicant), past experience with the relationship (e.g. old friends where one person is more dominant, older brother in relation to younger sister) or ability in the situation (e.g. being knowledgeable about cars versus ignorant when a car breaks down). Sometime status is overtly awarded (e.g. when a guest of honour is announced) but more often status is implicitly conferred or claimed by the way people interact. Social status is often communicated through subtle behaviours: we establish an unconscious structure of deference and social value. Status reflects who is in charge, and acknowledging their order in the social hierarchy keeps social relations stable and harmonious.

Within any group the social status of a person may change depending on the situation. For instance, for the duration of a team-building exercise the social status of the boss may be lowered and he may have equal status to the other team members during the exercise. Similarly, during family games adults become equal with the children for the duration of the game. Friends and relationships often have a balanced shifting of status depending on the situation and activity.

People with dementia almost always experience a loss of social status. They stop working and lose status associated with their work role. Socially, because of their loss of cognitive abilities, they are less able to make a contribution through work or conversation and lose status this way. Sometimes people with dementia are talked over or talked about as if they are not there, which further diminishes their status. If you have an established relationship with the person with dementia then you would also have your usual status roles. This may have changed since the person developed dementia. Reflect on this status, and whether you want to give the person with dementia greater status during some of your interactions with them.

I try to confer the people with dementia I interact with equal or higher status during our interactions. There are several ways in which I do this. Firstly, I use body language, bringing myself to the person's level, making eye contact, not taking up too much 'space'. I am attentive rather than dismissive. People with high status often look past rather than at those with lower status, as if they are not worthy of their full attention. People with higher status also tend to look down on those with lower status (e.g. a king on a throne) and take up lots of physical room.

Secondly, I ask the person with dementia their opinion and give them choice. People with high status tend to tell those of lower status what to do — for instance managers give instructions to their staff, fathers reprimand their children and doctors advise their patients. Rather than telling the person to do an activity, I ask what she thinks and offer her choices. I ask for permission to sit down and talk with her, I invite her to do activities with me,

I ask for her help. At the end of our interaction, I thank her for her time, tell her I enjoyed her company (if I did) and ask if I can talk with her again.

Thirdly, I give the person with dementia the chance to give back. Humans have evolved to be social creatures. Those of our ancestors who could cooperate better with their social group survived, possibly because they hunted better and defended themselves against predators better. Part of being social creatures is that we're compelled both publically and internally to be reciprocal in our behaviour, meaning that we're expected to help others who help us. Most of us feel that we need to repay favours, and failure to do so brings slight feelings of inadequacy or guilt. For instance, I feel guiltier forgetting the birthday of a friend who always remembers my birthday than forgetting the birthday of a friend who never remembers mine.

Some people with dementia feel they are a burden to their family and others, particularly because they are not contributing in any way. Giving people with dementia the chance to 'give back' evens up the social debt they may feel. To let the person with dementia give back, I may ask for their company for an activity, their advice during a conversation or their help in completing a task. This gives the activity/conversation/task added meaning because there is a social reason to do the task, i.e. fulfilling my request. I also acknowledge their contribution, listen to their advice, compliment their efforts, laugh at their jokes and enjoy their company. I appreciate what they have given back. We usually think of giving back as physically returning a favour, but giving back can also include returning positive energy and feelings and being generous in interactions with others.

PRESENTING ACTIVITIES FOR PERSONS WITH DEMENTIA

There are a number of things you can do before beginning the activity to increase your chances of success.

Prepare

Before you start, make sure you have all the equipment you will need for the activity and mentally rehearse what you are going to do.

For instance, if you are going on an outing, make sure that before you head out you have the address and location and have looked over a map, and you have keys and money, food and water if needed. It can also be useful to know whether there are toilets at your destination. If you are showing the person a book, look over the pages first and prepare some questions or comments to start the conversation. You may also have a back-up or alternative activity prepared.

Set the scene

Before trying to engage a person with dementia make sure he is comfortable. Is he hungry? Does he need to use the toilet? Is he in pain or feeling unwell? Make sure that his physical needs are attended to otherwise these concerns will reduce his ability to concentrate on you and the activity.

When you start talking to the person with dementia, make sure he can hear you and see you properly. Has he got his glasses or hearing aids on if he needs them? Sit on his 'good' side in terms of sight and hearing.

Minimize distractions. Switch off the television or radio. Clear the table if you are sitting at the table to do an activity. Make it easy for him to concentrate on you rather than spending energy blocking out competing information.

Connect with the person and invite them to participate in the activity

Make eye contact with the person with dementia, make sure you have their attention and say their name in greeting. Smile. I like to use the person's name frequently during our interaction; this keeps their attention and helps maintain rapport.

Unless you are sure that the person with dementia knows who you are, introduce yourself. Give your name as well as your relationship. If you simply say 'Hi Mum' they may not remember which child you are, or your name. Whereas if you say 'Hi Mum, it's Julie' then you've reoriented them to who you are.

Always give the person with dementia the choice to participate in the activity. In inviting the person to participate, think of why he might want to start the activity. Is the activity, at face value, of interest to him? Could he agree to start it because he likes doing something with another person? Could he agree to start it because he would like to help you?

Pitch your invitation based on the reason you think the person with dementia might participate in the activity. This may simply mean that you ask the person if they want to participate in the named activity, or if they want to participate in activity A or activity B (giving them choice at the same time). Alternatively you could ask the person for his help, or if he would like to do something together with you. Another approach is to engage him in conversation first to establish rapport and a relationship and then, when he seems to be in a receptive mood, invite him to participate in an activity together. Yet another approach is to start doing the activity where he can observe you and then invite him to join in after he has observed you — or he might even spontaneously join in. It is not usually a good tactic to ask the person to do the activity 'because it is good for you'. Many of us don't do things just because we have been told they are good for us.

If the person with dementia repeatedly refuses invitations to participate given through different approaches and for different activities, I would then reconsider the choice of activities, the invitation to participate and the person making the approach. Try to see if a different person, a different approach and different activities makes a difference and build from any small successes. A small success would be the person agreeing to participate in the activity, even if he quickly loses interest. In this context it would be worthwhile investigating and understanding any clinical causes of this resistance such as depression or chronic pain, or historical explanations such as a lifelong dislike of strangers.

Present the activity

During the activity provide appropriate support, monitor the person with dementia's response and modify the activity if needed; additionally, provide consistent positive feedback and follow his lead.

During the activity remember to use the communication strategies described earlier. Talk less and watch more. Watch and assess the person's reactions and interactions, and modify the activity accordingly. To modify the activity, use the principles of task analysis described in Chapter 3, such as taking away a step or providing more support. If you decide to abandon an activity, always offer an alternative activity that you can do together. You don't want to leave the person with dementia feeling as if you've left because they failed at the activity.

JUDGING THE SUCCESS OF AN ACTIVITY

Throughout your interactions with the person with dementia, observe her body language and facial expressions and let this guide your interactions. People with dementia have less control of their emotions and can be more unpredictable in their reactions, so we have to be extra aware of their mood when communicating with them.

The signs of engagement of someone with mild dementia may be obvious. However, I am often asked how to tell whether someone with severe dementia is engaged with and enjoying an activity. Below are some signs of interest and engagement for people with dementia.

Signs of engagement and interest

- Looking at you or the objects you are presenting — he or she may turn their head or lean forward or make eye contact.
- Nodding, clapping or responding in other ways.
- Talking — the words might not always be clear or make sense, but talking indicates they are responding to you.
- Touching, holding, approaching you or the object you are presenting.

The person with dementia may not follow an instruction or pick up an object but this does not mean they are not interested in interacting with you if the other signs of engagement are there. If you think the person has not attended to what you presented, you could either repeat it or try another approach.

Signs of disengagement, boredom or tiredness

- Looking away or down for a prolonged period.
- Getting up and moving away, leaning back, pulling away.
- Closing their eyes (except if appropriate, such as when listening to music or a story).

- Doing something else — the person may still want to interact with you but might not be interested in the activity or not understand what you want them to do.
- Talking about something else — the person may want to interact with you but might not be interested in the topic or might be unable to follow your conversation.

Signs of enjoyment
- Smiling, laughing.
- A peaceful or calm expression.
- An expression of concentration.

Signs of distress
- A grimace that is different from their usual expression.
- Angry, anxious or sad facial expressions.
- Talking about angry, scary or sad things.
- Aggressive behaviour towards you or the objects — e.g. throwing the object, yelling.

GIVE REGULAR, CONSISTENT, POSITIVE FEEDBACK

Activities sometimes have 'right' and 'wrong' responses or ways of doing things, but almost all the time it does not really matter whether the person with dementia's response is right or wrong. Even in a task where the outcome could be affected if they do the activity incorrectly, such as when making a cup of tea, it does not matter if the end product is not ideal.

Give regular, ongoing praise. Useful phrases include 'good work', 'well done', 'nice job', 'that's great', 'super' and 'thank you'. If the person has done something incorrectly, continue to use the same phrases in your feedback. If the person knows they've done it incorrectly or cannot do it correctly and becomes frustrated, encourage them to try again and support them to succeed. Say, 'That's okay, it is difficult, so let's do it together.'

FOLLOW THEIR LEAD

Sometimes when a person with dementia does something 'wrong', rather than ignoring it, this can be an opportunity to take the activity into a different direction than planned. For instance, you may have dealt the cards for a simple card game such as snap, but the person with dementia might instead start sorting the cards or building a card tower with the cards. Instead of bringing them back to the task of snap, go along with what the person wants to do and support them arranging the cards into suits or building the tower.

DEALING WITH STRONG NEGATIVE REACTIONS

A risk we take in any interaction with another person is that they could react negatively. It can be hurtful and upsetting if I've put time and effort into coming up with an activity and the person with dementia yells abuse at me or is violent in response.

Even if I've been watching carefully for warning signs such as restlessness, anxiousness or agitated behaviour, I might not have been able to predict the person with dementia was going to have a strong negative reaction. Or I might have noticed the signs but not been able to calm the person down and their behaviour has escalated.

If this occurs, firstly I try to stay calm. If there is any chance that I or someone else is in danger of being hurt, I reduce that risk by removing myself or the other people present or by getting help. Listen to what the person with dementia is saying, and watch what she is doing, and try to figure out what has made the person upset. If possible, I try to fix what has upset the person. Even if you can't figure out the cause, reassure the person and distract her. If more appropriate I give her space. If this happens to you, don't take it personally; remember that their reaction is not something you have control over, even if it directly occurred in reaction to your behaviour. It is really important to discuss the incident with someone else (debrief) afterwards. Reflect on what you would do differently in the future.

Often, the person with dementia will forget the incident and be happy to have your company again on another occasion. But be cautious when approaching the person the next time.

SELF-REFLECTION

Please think about your last few interactions with the person or people with dementia you care for. In the table opposite indicate the areas that you would like to improve, and then work on each skill until you are satisfied with your performance. Each time you present an activity it is also worthwhile briefly reflecting on how you have gone and what things you could improve the next time. Professional carers could include these reflections in their care notes.

SCHEDULING ACTIVITIES

It is a good idea to plan when you're going to present an activity. The timing may be based on certain times of the day when the person is likely to be in a better mood or have better attention or higher energy. You might also plan activities to meet the person's needs, for example if he tends to feel lonely after a visit from a friend or relative you could have an activity prepared for after that visit. Or you might choose a time when the person with dementia seems to have excess energy and be pacing or doing repetitive things, and give him an activity that lets him channel that energy, such as singing songs or going for a walk. Some people with dementia can sometimes be unpredictable in public, so you might want to bring an activity to engage them in situations where they may be bored such as in a doctor's waiting room.

Table 3: Areas for improvement

Skill or behaviour	I would like to improve on this
Watching the person with dementia more	
Watching my own mood more	
Watching my own behaviour more	
Matching my speed and intensity to theirs	
Talking less	
Choosing appropriate conversation topics	
Not arguing or correcting	
Giving the person with dementia status	
Giving the person with dementia choice	

Skill or behaviour	I would like to improve on this
Giving the person with dementia a chance to give back	
Preparing for the activity properly	
Making the initial connection	
Inviting them to participate in the activity	
Presenting the activity	
Modifying the activity	
Giving positive feedback	
Following the person with dementia's lead	
Dealing with strong negative reactions	

Activity calendars

It would be great for people with dementia to do a meaningful activity every day, and even several times a day. An activity calendar will help you plan activities and can be written into the existing family calendar or diary, or specifically drawn up. If multiple people are involved in the person's care, then an activity calendar will let everyone know what is happening, or has happened, for that person.

For family carers, writing out the calendar may seem like a lot of planning, however planning the activities means they are more likely to happen regularly and you don't need to think 'what next?' all the time. You can also see if there is a 'spread' of different types of activities. If you have a friend or paid carer come to care for the person with dementia to give you a break, then you can plan some activities they can do together. Having a regular activity schedule also provides a stimulating routine for the person with dementia. Activity planning on a monthly basis also gives you an opportunity to brainstorm new ideas for activities the person would like, based on your experiences of the previous month. Make the plans as tailored and specific as possible, and try to get a mix of activities that are cognitively stimulating, involve socialization and physical activity. And of course they should all be meaningful and achievable!

For professional carers, activities should form part of care plans, although I have rarely seen individualized activity plans. Tailoring activity calendars as much as possible (with the input of family caregivers and the person with dementia) will maximize the chance that the person will participate willingly, successfully and frequently. Nursing homes have the challenge of limited staff hours and resources when trying to cater for every individual resident. Nursing homes usually have activity programs for the whole facility or different sections of the facility, however since it is unlikely that many activities on this program are appropriate for the person with dementia, a personalized activity calendar would provide much better recreational care.

Examples of personalized activity calendars

On the following pages are some examples of what personalized activity calendars might look like for three of the people we are following in our case studies: Joy, Antonio and Ruth. In keeping with taking into account the thinking abilities of the person with dementia, note that it is likely to be more possible to plan a greater number and diversity of activities for the person with mild dementia than for those with greater cognitive impairment. People with dementia usually do not mind repeating activities they like.

Activity calendar for Joy (mild dementia, living at home)

	Monday	Tuesday	Wednesday	Thursday	Friday	Saturday	Sunday
Morning	Go for a walk; Joy to put out the laundry	Day outing – once a month Probus meeting, otherwise trip into the city or to art gallery or museum	Go for a walk	Grocery shopping	Social event either in the morning or afternoon, at least fortnightly. Otherwise visit local library or run other errands	Go for a walk to local park where children's sports teams play	Go for a drive, possibly have lunch out
Afternoon	Home activities*		Home activities*	Home activities*		Home activities*	Home activities*
Evening	Joy to set the table and they will cook dinner together	Joy to set the table and they will cook dinner together	Joy to set the table and they will cook dinner together	Joy to set the table and they will cook dinner together	Joy to set the table and they will cook dinner together	Go out for dinner, possibly with friends	Joy to set the table and they will cook dinner together

*Home activities are: looking at fashion magazines, listening and dancing to music, sorting out clothes for charity, discussing actors and actresses, doing gardening together (Joy waters and deadheads flowers).

Activity calendar for Antonio (mild to moderate dementia, living at home)

	Monday	Tuesday	Wednesday	Thursday	Friday	Saturday	Sunday
Morning		Visit Francesco in nursing home	Activity at home	Grocery shopping	Attend Italian senior citizen's club	Prepare dish for family lunch	Family lunch
Afternoon	Activity at home*	Activity at home*	Pick up Tony from school and spend time with him, Sofia will pick Tony up, sometimes may stay for dinner	Activity at home*		Activity at home*	Activity at home*
Evening	Antonio Jr to visit on the way home from work, may walk together	Walk with Maria		Walk with Maria	Maria goes to church group	Walk with Maria	Walk with Maria

*Activity at home could include conducting an inventory of the pantry, pricing items or looking over Brunswick Juventus memorabilia.

Activity calendar for Ruth
(moderate dementia, living in a nursing home)

	Monday	Tuesday	Wednesday	Thursday	Friday	Saturday	Sunday
Morning	Scheduled: craft. Ruth will not participate, offer her knitting	Scheduled: bingo. Ruth will not participate, offer her knitting	Scheduled: bus trip. Ruth likes to attend, though requires one-on-one attention	Scheduled: armchair travel. Ruth will not participate, offer her knitting	Scheduled: reminiscence. Ruth may look at photo album if given one-on-one attention. Once every fortnight Ruth's friend Helena visits	Scheduled: cooking. Ruth usually goes to children's house for lunch (Julie or Hannah)	Scheduled: mass. Ruth likes to attend, may want to leave part way through
Afternoon	Scheduled: chair exercise. Ruth will not participate. Julie usually visits after work	Scheduled: gardening. Ruth will not participate. Hannah usually visits after work	Scheduled: chair exercise. Ruth will not participate. Terrence usually visits after work	Scheduled: gardening. Ruth will not participate. Romano usually visits after work	Scheduled: walking group	Scheduled: Saturday drinks and sing along. Ruth may listen for a while	Ruth has family visitors (Julie or Hannah)

Ruth's calendar shows the group activities scheduled by the facility; however Ruth refuses or is cognitively not able to participate in most of these. The family compensate by visiting every day.

5

COGNITIVELY STIMULATING ACTIVITIES

What do you do that gives your brain a workout? I find that activities such as travel, attending a course or workshop or conference, meeting new people, going to a festival or parade, organizing a big event or performing on stage all work out my brain. What these activities have in common is that they require me to process and react to a lot of new information.

People with dementia often find it difficult to cope with a lot of new information. Most people with dementia would find it challenging, though not necessarily impossible, to travel, learn something new, meet many new people or go to a crowded event. This is why they are advised to keep to a routine and avoid potentially overstimulating experiences. However, there is a downside to sticking to a routine. Routines tend to reduce the opportunities to give their brain a workout. A stimulating routine is what we should aspire to create for people with dementia.

This chapter gives ideas about how to develop and deliver tailored cognitively stimulating activities for people with dementia. The 'dose' that has been shown to be beneficial in improving cognitive function for people with dementia is two 45-minute group sessions per week. Increasing the amount of cognitive activity may increase the positive impact, however this has not been shown. To achieve cognitive benefits, try to provide a minimum of 90 minutes of cognitively stimulating activity every week, spread out across as many sessions as needed. Conduct a range of different activities that exercise different aspects of thinking and memory. Most of the ideas discussed in the other chapters can be cognitively stimulating.

An engaging philosophy of care is cognitively stimulating. We encourage the person with dementia to think, experience and interact with different things every day. Choose issues or topics that the person finds interesting. Alternatively, use the social aspect of the activity to make the discussion meaningful. In general, ask for opinions rather than facts. When the person is asked to solve a problem, celebrate their achievements — do not point out their errors. If the person is unable to solve a problem by themselves, work together with them towards success.

What the science tells us

Researchers have tried three mental activity-based approaches to improve the cognitive abilities of people with dementia.

There is good consistent evidence for the benefits for cognition of cognitive stimulation therapy, which focuses on encouraging and facilitating fun and stimulating discussions. Cognitive stimulation therapy has the same benefits on maintaining cognitive functions as currently available drugs (e.g. cholinesterase inhibitors) for Alzheimer's disease. This is typically delivered in a small group of four to five people with mild to moderate dementia for 45 minutes, twice a week for fourteen weeks. Sessions have a set structure typically including introductions, discussion about day, season and current affairs, a song, a ball game, the main discussion topic for the day, summary and farewell. Examples of discussion topics may be famous faces, using money, word games and personal histories.

The benefits of cognitive stimulation therapy have been shown to be maintained for up to six months and it would be reasonable to assume that ongoing cognitive stimulation would provide ongoing benefit in slowing decline. The groups are led by a health professional, and detailed manuals are available for purchase (see 'Further resources', p. 230). Sessions aim to actively stimulate and engage people with dementia while providing an optimal learning environment and the social benefits of a group.

Cognitive training, or brain training, focuses on exercising specific mental abilities, such as short-term memory, attention or problem solving. The research has had mixed findings and overall brain training, either computerized or using pencil and paper, appears to improve the trained specific mental abilities, but does not lead to better general mental function or ability to do day-to-day tasks. This may be because brain-training exercises train a specific skill, such as remembering a list of words, and this skill doesn't generalize to other types of memory, such as remembering someone's name or remembering to watch a certain television show at a certain time. This is similar to how bicep curls don't improve leg strength or whole body strength.

Cognitive rehabilitation focuses on identifying and addressing individual cognitive difficulties. For instance, the person with dementia may want to learn the names of people in a group they attend, or to learn how to use a mobile phone. The therapist develops strategies to address their aims, using specific techniques for learning new information. Cognitive rehabilitation can help people with dementia address specific cognitive difficulties and maintain their daily functioning.

IDEAS FOR COGNITIVELY STIMULATING ACTIVITIES

Below are ideas for different types of cognitively stimulating activities for people with dementia. These do not have to be tightly tailored to the life history of a person with dementia. However, I would avoid topics they did not enjoy or were uninterested in earlier in life.

Treat all these ideas as springboards for conversation and discussion. The person with dementia should be stimulated to react to the topic or activity, to use their knowledge on the topic to generate an opinion and response, and communicate their thoughts or act on their response. While these activities have been described as being for one person, many would work very well in small groups. Treat this list as inspiration rather than prescription and create your own activities according to your situation.

Initiate a discussion or activity relating to the world, past or the present

This activity is more appropriate for people with mild to moderate dementia. Discussions should not just tap the person's knowledge about the topic but also their opinions and ideas. Activities may require the person to solve a problem, for instance using a map to plan a long-distance trip. Or the person might have to arrange three historical events in chronological order. Or they may have to answer true or false to a number of scientific 'facts'. You could think of these activities as similar to exercises that school students are given to encourage them to engage with a topic such as science, history or geography. However, where school students have to acquire knowledge as part of the task, the people with dementia use the knowledge they already have in the activity. Here are topics around which you can create discussions:

- the person's own life
- historical events
- famous people
- geography and places
- science
- current events
- politics and religion.

Do something creative or artistic focusing on the process, not the product

People with dementia often surprise us with what they create when given the opportunity. Perhaps it is because they are less inhibited due to changes in their frontal lobes. Perhaps it is because they live in the moment much more than those of us with better memories. Perhaps it is because they have fewer opportunities to express themselves. Whatever the reason, people with dementia have been shown to flourish when being artistic.

How do you get people with dementia to be creative? Give them some materials and some inspiration. Artists tell me that having a theme or focus stimulates rather than constrains creativity. A standard cognitive test requires a person with dementia to 'Write a sentence about anything you like'. We find that people with dementia find it difficult to think of a sentence to write. However, if we give that same person a photograph, and say 'Tell me a story about the person in this photograph' we find that they can make up many sentences worth of story. So, when presenting a creative activity, give the person a medium (e.g. storytelling or painting) and a theme to work on. Here are some further ideas:

- Storytelling: Use as a starting point a photograph, artwork, piece of music, video clip, smell or even food, or give an alternate ending to a story. A program called TimeSlips has shown how storytelling enables people with dementia to express themselves and connect with others (see 'Further resources', p. 230).
- Make visual art: Paint, draw, stick, colour, collage, sculpt. Themes could include 'If you had three wishes, what would they be?' or 'A day on the river' or 'Fruit'. You could encourage the person to observe something in real life and draw it, such as a still life or a landscape.
- Build something: Use craft materials or children's construction toys or Tupperware containers. You can suggest what you want them to build, such as a house or a tower.

Do something that stimulates the senses

Sensory stimulation can be very pleasurable, such as looking at a beautiful view. Discussion of sensory experiences in the moment can also stimulate other parts of the brain. Here are some ideas:

- Look at different pictures of art, then choose a favourite and explain why.
- Sing a song or make music (see Chapter 10 on music for more ideas).
- Taste test a range of different foods (e.g. fruit, biscuits or teas), scoring each one for appearance, taste and texture (or smell if tea) and choosing a favourite.
- Smell different scents (perfume, essential oil or food essences) and try to guess what they are, or talk about what they remind you of.

Play a game or do a puzzle

Choose games and puzzles on the basis that they are fun and encourage interaction rather than because they are mentally challenging. Try to avoid games that rely heavily on short-term memory. In general, don't be competitive about the game unless the person with dementia really wants to be competitive. You can also turn games traditionally played competitively or solitarily into a collaborative exercise. For instance, work together on a find-a-word or simple crossword (let the person with dementia do the circling or writing). Many children's games are also fun for people with dementia. It is possible to purchase larger versions of some games for older people with vision or manual dexterity difficulties. Here are some ideas for traditional games:

- snap
- pick up sticks
- Connect Four (also known as Four in a Line)
- magnetic fishing game
- dominoes
- I spy
- noughts and crosses
- picture bingo
- Scrabble or Boggle
- jigsaw puzzles (large size, fewer pieces).

Some books written specifically for people with dementia, for instance *Blue Sky White Clouds*, *The Sunshine on my Face* or the *Simple Pleasures for Special Seniors* series of books. Small inspirational books such as *The Blue Day Book* with short sayings and pictures may also be appropriate, as may be some books intended for children (as long as these are not too childish).

Here are some ideas for made-up games — you can also come up with your own!

- Guess the prices of objects taken out of the kitchen cupboard, or sort in order of cost.
- Choose items towards a purpose: For instance, choose items for a 'menu' for breakfast or lunch, or choose items for a toolbox, or presents for different family members. To make it more difficult, price the items and give the person a 'budget'.
- Word association games: Start by saying a word (e.g. banana). The next person says the next word they can think of relating to the first word (eat) and the next person says a word relating to the second word (cake). Write down the words if it helps the person with dementia follow what is happening. To make it harder, you could ask for all the words to start with a certain letter.
- Sorting category related games: If the person has the ability you could ask them to generate items for each category, otherwise get them to group items by category (e.g. countries of the world, bodies of water such as rivers versus seas, types of animals such as herbivores versus carnivores or farm animals versus zoo animals). The game can be played with words typed on paper, photographs or small objects (e.g. plastic animals). A simple version would be sorting items by colour or size (e.g. sewing cottons).

Experience and discuss nature

Do something that connects the person with the outside world. Being outdoors releases different chemicals in the brain than when indoors, and can improve stress levels and increase creativity. For example:

- Go for a walk and look for birds or other animals.
- Pat and interact with an animal.
- Feed the ducks at the local park.
- Look at the clouds and try to find animal shapes.
- Watch moving water.
- Explore by foot somewhere different.
- Go outside and look for objects of a certain colour (e.g. yellow).
- Collect objects (rocks, leaves, sticks, flowers, shells, pine cones) and arrange them in some way in the house to remind you of the experience (e.g. flower arrangement, small rock cairn, leaf collage).
- Play nature bingo — make a list of the things you're hoping to see when you're out on a walk, and try to tick them all off.

Discuss life's dilemmas

This activity works better with people with some verbal communication ability, as it relies on the person with dementia giving their opinion on a selected topic; it could, however, be adapted using pictures or objects for a person with dementia who doesn't speak well. Topics could be:

- Is a cat or dog a better pet?
- What kind of dog should I get as a pet?
- What is a good present for a child/60-year-old?
- Should I put in carpet or have floorboards?
- Should I go on holiday to the beach or the mountains?

Case study

JOY

Bernie has created some activities that he thinks may be cognitively stimulating for Joy, based on her interest in fashion and travel.

Bernie: 'Joy, I found these magazines in the garage and I wondered if you still wanted to keep them. Why don't you have a look through and see if you still want them?' (Bernie hands Joy two 30-year-old magazines)

Joy: 'Look at that lovely outfit. That colour suits her complexion.'

Bernie: 'Are there any outfits that you like? I've got some post-it notes here, maybe you could put a sticker on anything you really like.'

Joy: 'I like this black-and-white suit here. It's very smart.'

The conversation continued for a few minutes more, with Joy providing commentary on the outfits she liked. While this activity was of interest to Joy, it didn't sustain her attention for long and wasn't very cognitively difficult for her. Perhaps it lacked meaning or purpose for Joy as well. Bernie then developed a fashion-related sorting activity for Joy and tried it a few days later.

Bernie: 'Joy, I've got some pages out of fashion magazines and I was wondering if you could help me sort them. I'd like your opinion on which outfit would be good for work, which would be good for weekends, and which are evening wear.'

Joy: 'This is a lovely dress. I wouldn't mind one of those.'

Bernie: 'Is it for work, for weekends or evening wear?'

Joy: 'Evening wear. Maybe with a long string of pearls and a little jacket.'

Bernie: 'Great.' (places it on the evening-wear pile, hands her another picture)

Joy: 'I don't like that so much.'

Bernie: 'Is it for work, for weekends or evening wear?'

Joy: 'For weekends, but I wouldn't wear it.'

Bernie: 'Great. Can you put it here on the weekend pile? Take another picture.'

Joy: 'That's a work suit. With pants, not a skirt.'

Bernie: 'Thanks. The work pile is here.'

Joy: (places the picture on the pile, then picks up another picture) 'A pencil skirt and white blouse. That's for work.' (places it on the evening-wear pile)

Bernie: (ignoring Joy's mistake) 'Great.'

The activity continued with Joy sorting the clothing pictures into piles. Bernie used the same question each time in this activity, and after a few pictures Joy didn't require the question. He doesn't correct Joy when she makes a mistake. There were opportunities for the conversation to take a different direction; for instance, after Joy said that she wouldn't wear an outfit Bernie could have asked what she didn't like about it or why she wouldn't wear it. Bernie could have experimented with how much prompting or gesturing he needed to give Joy, or whether she could do the activity with minimal assistance. Also, the next time they do the activity Joy may need even less prompting (even if she doesn't remember ever doing the activity before).

A few days later, Bernie tries an even more challenging activity with Joy — storytelling.

Bernie: 'Joy, I was clearing out this cupboard and I found some old postcards.'

Joy: 'Oh, these are from England and France.'

Bernie: 'Yes, I can't remember when we bought them.'

Joy: 'I don't think we bought them. Someone must have given them to us.'

Bernie: 'Could be. But they are blank. Do you want to pretend that we're on holiday and write them to someone?'

Joy: (looks blank)

Bernie: 'Let's try it. Let's pretend that we're in England on holiday in the Cotswolds.'

Joy: 'That sounds good.'

Bernie: 'What shall we say?'

Joy: 'I don't know.'

Bernie: 'How about we tell them what we've been doing on holiday in England?'

Joy: 'Yes, let's say we're having a great time

even though it's been raining.'

Bernie: 'Okay. You write that down.' (Joy writes the
            sentence down)

Joy: 'Now what?'

Bernie: 'What shall we say we've been doing?'

Joy: 'Driving through the countryside?'

Bernie: 'That sounds good ... write that ...'

Joy: 'How about that we've been driving past
            hedgerows and robins? They have lots of
            those here in England.'

Bernie: 'Good idea ... write that.'

The conversation continues until the postcard is full, then
they write a postcard from France.

PRACTICAL TIPS

Develop a mentally stimulating routine. Take
and make opportunities to do things that
encourage the person with dementia to think.
Thinking doesn't just mean doing puzzles
or maths; it could be scrutinizing the world
around them (e.g. birdwatching), making
something (e.g. craft, cooking), discussing
abstract ideas (e.g. talking ethics or religion),
solving problems (e.g. checking the monthly
budget) and working things out (e.g. planning a
holiday). Try to exercise different functions of
the brain discussed in Chapter 2.

You might want to protect the person with dementia from doing mentally challenging activities in case they fail or get upset at their performance. Avoidance of more difficult tasks may protect their self-confidence or make them feel as if you don't think they are capable of doing them. If the person is protected from mentally challenging activities they will probably exercise their brain less, and also lose opportunities to socialize and do some things they might enjoy.

When the person with dementia is doing mentally challenging activities, maximize their chances of success by modifying the activity and supporting the person with cues and prompts as described in Chapter 3.

Plan the day so that the person is doing cognitively stimulating activities at a time when they are at their best. For instance, plan to do these activities mid-morning if that is when they are most alert. Or if you have an evening engagement, plan a quiet day so that the person has more mental energy at night.

There is a myth that people with dementia can no longer learn new things. People with dementia can and do learn new things; however, this can take longer and be more effortful. There are specific techniques used in cognitive rehabilitation with people with mild dementia that may help with specific information that the person with dementia wants or needs to learn.

Learning procedures

Motor and procedural memories are encoded and stored separately to memories for facts and events. Take tying a shoe lace. You know the movements of how to tie a shoe lace. However, if I asked you to write down how to tie a shoe lace you would have to think about it, because the process is stored in motor memory, not in words. The memory systems for procedures tend to be less affected by dementia, particularly Alzheimer's disease, than memory systems for facts. So, when teaching someone with dementia a procedure, don't give a list of consecutive instructions — rather, train the motor movements. Practise doing the sequence with the body and objects. For instance, if the person with dementia needs to learn how to turn on a new television, don't just give the instruction, 'Press the green button on the remote'. Give the person the remote control, point at the green button and get them to press it as you explain. Then repeat the procedure until they have learnt it.

Learning the names of people

The more a person thinks about and processes information when trying to learn it, the more likely they are to remember it. One way of adding processing is to think about the information in a different way. So, if the person is trying to learn someone's name, instead of just repeating the name 'Adam, Adam, Adam' to them, you can add the description, 'Adam, he was the first man in the creation story, he was tempted by the apple. Can you picture Adam eating an apple?'

You can prepare a photo album of people with their names, that the person can use to refresh their memory of people's names.

Another technique for learning new information is to practise recalling or retrieving the information from storage within a short time of learning it, when more likely to remember it. So, within an hour of learning the person's name you might try prompting the person with dementia to remember the name again, and then prompt them to practise remembering it again within 2 hours, then 5 hours, then 10 hours and then 24 hours, extending the time between practices. This technique is called spaced retrieval, because you space out the delay between retrieving the memory each time. Every time the person's name and face are remembered they are also being more firmly written into the memory banks.

Method of loci

The method of loci is a technique for remembering lists of things in a certain order. The technique involves choosing a physical route that is known well, such as the walk from your bedroom to the lounge room, or the walk from your house to church. As you walk the route in your mind, you associate each landmark (the bed, the cupboard, the bedroom door, etc.) with an item on your list. You mentally practise walking the route until you've learnt the associations. When you need to remember the list, you can then walk the route in your mind and use each landmark as a prompt.

6

REMINISCENCE

In a nutshell, reminiscence involves encouraging a person with dementia to talk about their past and making them feel good through remembering and sharing. Reminiscence is, by definition, meaningful. You can help make it achievable by stimulating the reminiscence, encouraging more recall and helping the person with dementia through any difficulties with expressing themselves. Many older people, particularly people with dementia, seem to live in the past, so to get them to reminisce is often easy. I will share some skills and tips that may elicit a greater range of reminiscences and increase how good the person feels after sharing those memories.

WHAT IS REMINISCENCE?

All of us think back through our past experiences. These memories remind us who we are and sometimes give us ideas for how to deal with the future. Reminiscence does not usually involve just remembering the details of events from the past. It often also involves re-experiencing the feelings associated with the experience, and reflecting on it, such as by commenting on what was learnt from the experience, or the difference between the past and today. Sometimes as we remember an event we re-evaluate or even rewrite the experience, we analyze and interpret the memories and process with hindsight.

For instance, when I think back on my childhood I remember happy visits to my grandparents' house. My grandmother did patchwork and was always busy turning fabric scraps and old clothes into beautiful blankets. My grandfather did all the cooking and would always make my favourite dish, roast duck soup. I particularly adored my grandfather, who would always buy treats and was a great storyteller. These memories reinforce that I come from a creative family and that I am much loved. As an adult I learnt that my grandfather was a lady's man. This made me re-evaluate my memories of him, and particularly made me remember my grandmother and her kindness and love for my grandfather in a different light.

People with dementia are forced to shift from being drivers and controllers of their world to being more passive. It may be that remembering occasions when they were an active participant helps maintain their self-worth and integrity. Just having someone spend time listening to their stories will reinforce the feeling that the person has worth. By listening, we are placing value on the person's life and experiences. Indeed, studies have shown that reminiscence therapy improves mood, wellbeing and aspects of cognitive function in people with dementia.

People who spend a lot of time at home (or in a nursing home) can escape the relative monotony of their lives through recalling past experiences. Many older people start to think that they are nearing the end of their life, and in this context it is often important for them to reflect on the life they have lived and the legacy they are leaving behind, and to feel that their life had meaning.

We store strongly emotional memories much better than memories without emotions attached to them. This is because strong emotions are usually associated with either highly positive or highly negative events. In both cases we remember those events in order to better repeat or avoid them in the future. Because of this, events that produced a strong emotion are usually recalled more often and in greater clarity and detail than non-emotional events. Interestingly, the mood we are currently feeling affects the memories we recall; we are more likely to remember events associated with moods matching our current moods than events associated with other moods. So, someone who is depressed is more likely to remember bad, sad events from their past, whereas someone who is happy is more likely to recall previous positive occasions.

Life review reminiscence is a structured therapeutic technique used by trained clinicians. The conversation begins with the individual's earliest memory and progresses to the present. The clinician asks probing questions in an attempt to elicit deepest thoughts and secrets, both positive and negative, and to assist the person to experience their feelings and significance of past events. Life review reminiscence also attempts to resolve regrets and past conflicts. This type of reminiscence therapy may not be enjoyable during the conversation, even though the end result may be improved mental health. I do not suggest that untrained carers try life review reminiscence.

Simple reminiscence consists of the person recalling past memories in a less structured way than life review reminiscence. There is a greater emphasis on reminiscence being a pleasant experience, and less emphasis on working through past issues. The key is not just remembering the memories, but having someone to listen, empathize with and share the experiences.

THERE ARE RISKS TO REMINISCENCE

The person with dementia may become distressed through recalling painful memories. You might know the topics from the person's past that could upset them and are better avoided such as wartime experiences or the loss of a family member. However, some people have processed their painful past experiences and can remember them with sadness but without a strong catastrophic reaction. You might not know all the topics from the person's past, though, and might unknowingly cause them to recall a memory that is extremely painful; if this occurs, reassure them and keep them calm. I will give specific examples about how to do this in the section titled 'Active listening' (p. 133).

The person with dementia may reveal a secret that might have implications for the family, such as that one of the children was adopted into the family or a baby was adopted out of the family, or that abuse occurred in the past. If this happens, decisions would also need to be made about who to tell. The person with dementia should be consulted about what he or she wants in regard to such secrets.

Talking about a negative past experience is not necessarily to be avoided if the person with dementia wants to reminisce about it. Some people have dealt with negative events and are not highly emotionally affected by their recall, and may value talking about how they have resolved the issues. Some people also seem to enjoy sharing and gaining sympathy from past experiences.

HOW TO DO SIMPLE REMINISCENCE

There are several ways to encourage people with dementia to talk about the past. The life history of the person will give you hints about what objects or topics may stimulate reminiscence. To start the reminiscence you could ask questions, discuss photographs and objects relating to the person's past, or even visit places relating to the person's past. If you're getting to know the person, use pieces of information you gather from one conversation to select objects and questions for the next session. The library and internet are great sources of information and stimuli. Old photographs of the places the person knew (town, school, landmarks), old magazines from the country and period, recipe books from the country and period, tourism guide books or brochures about significant places, and historical books can all trigger memories and start conversations. Often objects in the person's home are also a great starter of reminiscence such as family photos, handicrafts, ornaments or artworks. Music can also trigger memories, as can other sounds (for more on selecting music see Chapter 10). Smells and food are other powerful triggers of memories, particularly of emotions; however, these are more difficult to use as stimuli.

If you're going to use questions to elicit reminiscence, start with an open question. An open question is a question likely to produce a long answer, one that allows the person to choose what they want to talk about and invites them to discuss their opinions and feelings. Open questions give the person with dementia control of the conversation and also allow them to recall memories that they can access. Here are examples of open questions that you could ask to start the conversation:

- 'Tell me about your childhood.'
- 'What did you do for a job?'

- 'What was your first job like?'
- 'What did you do for fun when you were younger?'
- 'Did you travel?' followed by 'What was that like?'
- 'How did you meet your husband/wife?'
- 'Tell me about your children.'

In contrast, closed questions can be answered in a single word or short phrase, and try to elicit a specific fact. Closed questions leave the control of the conversation with the person asking the question. Closed questions are less likely to get someone talking, and are more likely to upset a person with dementia because they cannot remember a specific piece of information. Examples of closed questions that I do not recommend using during reminiscence include: 'When were you born?' 'What are the names of your grandchildren/old pets/old company?'

Case study

ANTONIO

Sofia has come to spend time with Antonio. She feels it is important they spend time together before his condition deteriorates.

Sofia: 'Papa, how are you?'

Antonio: 'Bene, bene, grazie.'

Sofia: 'Papa, I want to write down some stories about your life in Italy before you came to Australia so that I can share them with Tony. Have you got any old photos of you in Italy?'

Antonio: 'Si.' (He looks for the photos, and with Maria's help gets out an old shoe box of photographs.)

Sofia: 'Oh, I haven't seen these photos in years. Tell me about this one.'

Antonio: 'This is me. And this is my mother, Bianca.'

Sofia: 'I wish I could have met her.'

Antonio: 'She was an angel. She did everything for us. Cooking, cleaning. She cooked everything fresh. No tinned or packet food. She made sure our clothes were perfectly ironed and clean every day, all six of us.'

Sofia: 'Did Bianca ever go out and work?'

Antonio: 'No, no, her work was looking after us. She sewed most of our clothes, looked after the house, vegetables and animals. She used to say that we were her little treasures.'

Sofia: 'What animals did you have?'

The conversation continues for quite a while with Antonio reminiscing about the past ...

Sofia: 'Sounds like life was much harder when you were growing up than it is now, Papa?'

Antonio: 'Yes, nowadays everyone has so much money, but they are so busy. They don't have time for family like before.'

Sofia: 'I have time for you and Mamma.'

Antonio: 'Yes, you always come and see us.'

Sofia: 'Thank you for telling me your stories.'

Antonio: 'Thank you, thank you.'

This example is an illustration of how easily some older people reminisce. Sofia may have heard many of the stories before, but Antonio would not have remembered this, and enjoyed telling them.

ACTIVE LISTENING

Once the person with dementia has started reminiscing, encourage them to keep talking and make sure they feel listened to. Active listening skills can help with this.

Perhaps you are already a naturally good listener. Active listening skills will improve your listening skills and are used by clinicians such as psychologists, counsellors and social workers. These skills are also being increasingly taught to sales people because of how they can be used to enhance building of rapport and understanding of the other person. The skills are designed to make the person talking feel heard and encouraged to keep talking; they also validate their experiences and feelings.

Clinicians use some active listening techniques with people in therapy to help their patients explore and process their experiences and feelings, but we do not need to do this for simple reminisce. I've included skills here that I find useful when listening to a person with dementia, particularly when their ability to express themselves is difficult. The skills help us focus on the meaning of what the person is telling us, not just the details. Using these skills make us process the person's story more deeply. The phrases I suggest can also be helpful when you don't know what to say, for instance when someone tells you something very sad, or surprising, or shocking. When you read them on paper, these phrases might seem artificial or constructed, but I encourage you to try them — they work! You might also find some of these techniques useful during other life conversations, such as when talking with a friend going through a difficult break-up, when chairing a meeting or even when getting to know a stranger at a party.

Here are some active listening techniques:

Watch your own body language

This subject has already been covered but it is so important it is worth repeating. When listening, leaning forward shows interest although this can also be perceived as threatening; leaning back shows less interest. A neutral position is a good starting point. Crossed arms and legs can suggest defensiveness or a barrier to communication. Touching someone on the shoulder, forearm or top of the hand can often be reassuring or comforting. Nod a lot while the person is speaking and make good eye contact. This encourages a person to talk.

Let the person speaking control the conversation

Normal conversations are usually reciprocal, an exchange between two people. During reminiscence, leave control of the conversation and the focus of the conversation with the person with dementia. Let the person talk without trying to add your story or your opinion. If appropriate, you can briefly share your experience on a related topic or answer a question related to yourself, but do not take over the focus of the conversation. Some people with dementia become less interested in other people's lives and many lose interest altogether if you talk too much about yourself.

Invite the person to continue talking

This can be done by asking open questions. Phrases such as 'So what happened then ...' 'What was it like ...' 'Tell me more about ...' are useful in encouraging greater reminiscence without asking a more specific question.

Paraphrase and reflect back

It is helpful to paraphrase what the person with dementia has told you and then reflect it back to them. This shows them that you were listening and interested. To do this, you have to figure out the big picture from the details of their story. Paraphrasing means summarizing your interpretation of what they have told you in one or two sentences; reflecting means naming the feeling that the person was describing. I like to start my summary with phrases such as 'Sounds like this happened ...' or 'I'm hearing that ...' to show that it is my interpretation of what they have said in case I have misunderstood, instead of just stating my interpretation as if it is a fact. By giving the summary as if it is my opinion, it gives the person the opportunity to correct me or clarify the issue further. Here are some examples of paraphrasing:

- 'Sounds like your first job set you up for life.'
- 'What a wonderful story about your dog Charlie. Sounds like he really was important in your life.'

Here are some examples of reflecting:

- 'Sounds like you had a very happy childhood.'
- 'I'm hearing that there has been a lot of sadness in your life.'

Validate the person's experiences and feelings

Validation means showing that you have heard and accept the person's experiences and feelings. Validation is particularly useful when the person with dementia talks about a painful or difficult experience. If you tell them not to worry, or not to cry, or minimize the effect of the experience, it could seem to the person with dementia that you are minimizing their feelings. To accept a person's experience, you have to be prepared to listen to and share the feelings of sadness or anger that the person is expressing, and do this even though it makes you feel uncomfortable.

It can be helpful to summarize or reflect back on the painful experience, if possible adding a positive comment about the person (not the experience).

The following phrases may be useful:

- 'Sounds like a difficult situation.'
- 'Sounds like a very painful experience.'
- 'Sounds like it was a hard time.'
- 'Sounds like it was very difficult.'

A positive comment could be something like:

- 'You did well coming through that experience.'
- 'I'm impressed at what you survived.'
- 'You were very brave to have done that.'
- 'You coped very well given the circumstances.'
- 'You got through it, even though it was hard.'

DO NOT EXPECT PEOPLE WITH DEMENTIA TO BE ACCURATE HISTORIANS

Don't expect people with dementia to be good historians. They will not be consistent with their story from one reminiscence session to the next or even within the one session. They will provide information that does not make sense, they will provide information that you know is wrong. Do not question inconsistencies or correct them — if they recall something incorrectly it does not matter for the activity.

Do not try to keep the person with dementia on track or on topic. If they stray from the discussion topic at hand then let them talk about the topic they are interested in.

HELPING THEM FIND THE WORDS (SOMETIMES)

Sometimes a person with dementia becomes frustrated, annoyed or gives up trying to communicate because they can't remember the word or can't explain what they want to tell you. Try to minimize their frustration by helping them find the word, or by paraphrasing or reflecting what you've understood so far. Give them lots of positive feedback and encouragement, and don't express any frustration at how long they are taking or how difficult it is to understand what they are saying.

Case study

JOY

In the example below, Bernie encourages Joy to reminisce.

Bernie: 'Joy, look what I found while I was tidying out the cupboard.'

Joy: 'Video tapes.'

Bernie: 'Yes, video tapes of you on screen. Shall we watch them?'

Joy:	'No, no. That was when I was young and beautiful. I'm past that now.'
Bernie:	'But don't you want to just watch them and remember the times on set? Like the scene you did with Olivia Newton-John?'
Joy:	'Olivia. She was so friendly and nice. I remember she would drink tea on set and lots of water, and she hardly seemed to eat at all. She was always friendly with the extras. I said to her, "Olivia, can I ask you how your skin is always so perfect?" And she looked at me and said, "Drink lots of water and use the best products you can afford." Then she smiled that gorgeous smile. She was more beautiful in real life than on screen.'
Bernie:	'You've always talked fondly about Olivia. Who were other actors you liked?'
Joy:	'I don't know. There were lots of nice people.'
Bernie:	'How about Rolf Harris?'
Joy:	'Rolf Harris. I found him rather strange. He kept forgetting his lines and we had to do the scene over and over and over and over. It was quite funny the first few times. He wasn't bothered by it, though. I remember he had this big black bag that he would bring onto set full of musical instruments, and during the breaks he would sometimes get them out and sing a song. (sings) Tie

me kangaroo down, sport, tie me kangaroo
down ...'

(Bernie sings the rest of the song with Joy.)

Bernie: 'What's another Rolf Harris song? "Six
           white boomers".'

Joy: 'Six white boomers ... six white boomers
           ... la la la la la ... oh I can't remember
           the words. I know, I'll sing you another
           Christmas carol. Silent night, holy night ...'

Bernie had intended to watch old video tapes with Joy to
stimulate old memories and conversation, but she didn't
want to watch them and Bernie respected that choice.
Joy did briefly reminisce based on Bernie's questioning,
and his detailed knowledge of her past helped with this.
Joy then started singing and Bernie went along with
that rather than directing the conversation back to
reminiscence. Note that the one closed question that
Bernie asks about which other actors Joy liked didn't work
well because Joy couldn't remember the answer.

LIFE STORY WORK

Life story work involves documenting the life history of a
person with dementia. The product is a celebration of the life
of the person with dementia. Often the process helps the person
doing the documentation get to better know and understand
the person with dementia. The product of life story work can
then be used for future reminiscence and to help professional
carers understand the person and provide more person-centred
care. Life story work can also help the family of the person with

dementia find out information about their family history before those memories are lost. Life stories can be documented in different ways. There are commercially available books with a template to be filled in (see 'Further resources', p. 230). The life story can be typed up on a computer or written into a notebook. Life story work can also take the form of a series of audio or video recordings, an annotated photo album or a memory box of notated important objects from the person's life.

I wrote earlier that we cannot expect people with dementia to be accurate historians and that this does not matter during simple reminiscence. However, this may matter during life story work where the product is to be kept as a family record or used as a resource for professional care staff. Nonetheless, it is still not helpful to correct a person with dementia, or point out inconsistencies or repeatedly question details. Any details that are questionable should be corroborated, or an indication that the detail may not be accurate can be recorded.

Many people like to approach life story work chronologically, starting from early childhood and proceeding to the present day. While this is easier for the person documenting the story, it might not be as enjoyable for the person with dementia and may not be practically possible. Our memories are not stored chronologically and sometimes the pieces may emerge in non-ordered fashion. For instance, a discussion of the person's wedding might bring up stories about their best man who until this point had not been mentioned. A theme that continues throughout a person's life could be documented together, such as travel or an interest. Keep a folder with separate sheets for each story or with the notes for video, audio, photographs and objects. When they have been collected they can be arranged to best tell the person's story.

When writing the life history, write in the person's own words as much as possible. 'I was born in ...', 'My parents were called ...' etc. Here are topics that can be covered in a life story document:

- family life in childhood
- school days including friends and teachers, favourite subjects and achievements
- work life including first job, favourite job, interesting workplace anecdotes
- how they met spouse and wedding
- children from babyhood to adulthood
- pets
- cars
- celebrations such as significant birthdays, Christmas, New Year's Eve or other cultural festivals like Chinese New Year
- travel
- food loved and shared
- hobbies including craft, sports played or teams supported
- religion.

Life story work does not have to cover all these topics or provide a detailed, comprehensive historic record.

REMINISCENCE FOR PEOPLE WITH MODERATE TO SEVERE DEMENTIA

Research has shown that people with moderate and severe dementia can and do reminisce. However, their memories might be more fragmented and they may find it more difficult to describe these memories. The person listening will need to listen and respond more attentively so that the person with dementia's efforts at communication are successful, as this will encourage further engagement and reminiscence.

Memory aids have been shown to help people with moderate to severe dementia stay on topic and talk more during reminiscence. When trying to get the person with dementia to reminisce, provide them with items that they can see, touch and manipulate rather than having to keep the topic in their working memory. Further, if you give someone with dementia a few related stimuli on a topic, it will help them better recall information from their memory about that topic and can generate greater thinking and discussion on that topic.

Take the topic of weddings. Asking 'What was your wedding like?' gives one auditory clue, 'wedding', that might trigger recall of some ideas about weddings stored in the person's memories. Hearing the words marriage, white dress, vows and celebrations gives us more auditory cues that can trigger recall of more ideas relating to weddings. Listening to the reading of traditional wedding vows may stimulate yet different ideas, such as the episodic memory of a wedding that she has attended. Looking at photographs of weddings may bring up yet other ideas about weddings, as might touching and manipulating objects related to weddings such as an invitation, order of service, wedding rings in a box or decorated candles.

Case study

BRIAN

Gary and June have brought an old family photo album in an attempt to improve their visits with Brian. Brian is in his switched-off mode when they arrive but is eventually persuaded to open his eyes and look at the album. He turns a few pages then seems to enjoy looking at the few photographs of himself and his family when they were children. June, Gary's wife, talks to him:

(Brian touches the face of his mum in a photograph, says 'Mum' and seems sad.)

June: 'Is that your mum?'

Brian: 'Yes, Mum.'

June: 'Tell me about your mum.'

(Brian doesn't say anything, continues to pat the picture of his mum's face)

June: 'What was your mum's name?'

Brian: (after a long pause) 'Doris ... lovely.'

June: 'I'm sure she was a lovely mum, Do you love your mum?'

Brian: 'Yes, lovely ... lovely.'

June (pointing): 'Who is this with your mum?'

Brian: (pointing) 'Me.' (pointing) 'Richard.'

June: 'Who is Richard?'

Brian: (pointing) 'Richard.'

June: 'Is Richard your brother?'

Brian: 'Yes. Brother Richard.'

June: 'Where was this photo taken?'

Brian starts to turn the pages of the album again; he seems to spend time looking at the photos showing his childhood and the countryside. June continues to ask him questions, to which he sometimes gives answers. June also comments on the photographs. They sit and look at photographs for 10 minutes before Brian closes the album and pushes it away. June then says, 'Thank you for looking at those photos with me. Shall I bring photos again next time we come?' Brian nods.

The example above shows how using a stimulus (in this case a photograph) can help generate reminiscence. Brian may not have attended to or responded to June's conversation if she had just talked about his past. June followed Brian's lead by observing carefully which photographs he seemed more interested in and discussing those photographs rather than the photographs she was more curious about or that were interesting to her. The conversation and activity came to a natural end. For June and Gary the interaction made their visit more meaningful. Let's pick up the story at Gary and June's next visit to Brian.

Case study

BRIAN

Gary and June are pleased they have had some positive interactions with Brian. The next visit, they bring more old pictures of Brian and his family. Brian has been pacing up and down the corridor and trying to open all the locked doors. Gary says hello, and Brian pushes past him. 'Here we go again ...' says Gary, who turns to go and sit in the lounge. 'Let me try,' offers June. She takes out the photograph of Brian, Richard and their mother that Brian reacted to last visit. She holds it out and approaches

Brian, who is trying to open a door. 'Brian ... Brian ... here is a photograph of you and Richard and your mum.' She offers Brian the photo and he takes it. June comes to stand next to him to look at it.

June: (pointing) 'Is this your mum, Brian?'

Brian: 'Yes.'

June: (pointing) 'Is this you, Brian?'

Brian: 'Yes.'

June: 'You all look happy in this picture.'

Brian: 'Yes.'

June: (holding open photo album) 'Would you like to look at more photos?'

Brian: (looks at album for a while) 'No.' (He keeps looking at the photo in his hand.)

June: 'Let's sit down and look at that photo together.' (She takes Brian's arm, Brian follows her down the corridor and they sit down together.)

June: 'Let's see if there are any other photos of you and Richard and your mum. Here is one.' (hands it to Brian)

Brian: 'That's Mum.'

June: 'Yes, and that's you with a dog.'

Brian: 'Good dog.'

June: 'Do you like dogs?'

Brian: 'Yes, yes. They are good. Good dogs.'

Brian and June continue to look at and comment on the photos for a few more minutes before Brian gets up and starts pacing again.

June and Gary make a request that when the pet therapy dog visits, the staff trial a visit with Brian. Staff report that Brian responds well to the dog visits and they try to ensure he is able to spend time with the dog on future visits.

The above example shows how a person (June) and stimulus (photograph) can temporarily change the behaviour of a person with dementia. June had to get Brian's attention and gently but assertively invite him to look at the photos with her. It also shows how conversations and activities can generate new ideas about what the person might like. It showed June and Gary how they could still 'reach' Brian. Incidentally, researchers have found that people with mild to moderate dementia symptoms show enhanced mental health and physical function when interacting with dogs.

Let's now return to Brian's story a year later.

Case study

BRIAN

Brian's dementia has deteriorated and he no longer is able to talk, walk or control his hands very well. His personality seems to have shut down and he spends most of his time asleep, even when he is wheeled out into the common area. He seems to be awake only when being cared for or being fed. His nephews Gary and Daniel feel the end is near. However, June feels that they need to stimulate Brian even more and wants to keep connecting with 'the person inside the shell'.

On her next visit June brings with her a collection of different items that may be interesting to Brian: some locks of sheep wool, a horseshoe, a bag of hay and an old photograph of him and his mum. She sits down next to Brian and makes eye contact.

June: 'Here is a horseshoe.' (She gives him the
            horseshoe. He lifts it up so that he can see
            it. Then he drops his hands.)

June: 'Here is some clean hay.' (June puts the bag
            on Brian's chest and places his hands in the
            bag. Brian touches the hay for a while with
            his fingers, before again lifting some up to
            look at it. He looks at June.)

June: 'Hay, hay from a field.'

June: 'Brian, Uncle Brian, it's June, your niece.'
            (June takes hold of Brian's hand, Brian
            slowly opens his eyes, looks past June.)

June: 'How are you? You look well. Are you hot
            with so many blankets on? I'll take one off
            for you.' (Brian slowly closes his eyes again.)

June: 'Brian, I've brought some things for you to
            look at.' (June places the sheep wool in his
            hands.) 'Here is some sheep wool. It was
            only shorn last week.' (Brian's fingers slowly
            touch the wool and his trembling hands lift
            it up so that he can see it.)

June:	'Smell it, it smells of farm.' (Brian keeps looking and fingering the wool, and June helps him lift it to his nose. Brian takes one sniff and then another. His eyes open a little wider and he looks at June.)
June:	'It's merino. Very soft.' (Brian takes another sniff and then his fingers work the locks, trying to tug and pull them apart. He does this for a minute or so. Then he stops and looks at June.)
June:	(starts singing) 'There's a track winding back to an old-fashioned shack along the road to Gundagai. Where the gum trees are growin' and the Murrumbidgee's flowin' beneath the starry sky ...' (Brian nods his head and moves his hand along to the music, maintaining eye contact with June the whole time.)
June:	'Did you like that song?' (After a pause, Brian slowly nods and slowly blinks his eyes.)
June:	'Would you like to hear it again?' (Brian slowly nods.)
June:	(starts singing) 'There's a track winding back to an old-fashioned shack along the road to Gundagai. Where the gum trees are growin' and the Murrumbidgee's flowin' beneath the starry sky ...' (Brian closes his eyes while nodding to the music. June then takes out the photograph and puts it in Brian's hands.)

June: 'Brian, look at this.' (Brian brings the photo
          up to look at it. His face breaks into a weak
          smile. He looks at June.)

June: (pointing) 'Brian and Mum.' (Brian taps the
          faces on the photo, then brings it to his lips
          to kiss it.)

June: 'You love your mum.' (Brian slowly smiles.)

The above example shows how people with severe dementia
can derive enjoyment from simple sensory activities (looking at,
touching and smelling things, music) and can communicate and
respond non-verbally. I believe that it is important to provide
pleasure and connectedness for people no matter their abilities.

7

FRIENDS AND FAMILY

The saying traditionally goes that it takes a village to bring up a child. I believe that it takes a village to care for an elder. The more people involved in the life of the person with dementia, the more opportunities they have to be stimulated, to interact and engage, and the more people there are to emotionally support and love them and remind them of who they are.

FRIENDSHIPS ARE IMPORTANT

Think about your friendships and what they mean to you.

People with more or better quality friendships live longer, have better mental health, better physical health and are more resilient, meaning that they cope better with life's adversities. But despite their importance, we don't always put as much effort into developing and maintaining friendships as we do in maintaining physical health or economic security. Friends let us be ourselves and support us to become who we want to be. For someone with dementia, these aspects of friendship are very important.

DEMENTIA OFTEN BRINGS LOSS OF FRIENDSHIPS

As people get older, their social networks tend to become smaller. Some friends move away, others become sick, frail and less sociable, and sadly some pass away. Physical health, mobility and transport make it more difficult to see existing friends. Children and grandchildren seem to have busy lives and may live far away.

On top of all the changes to social networks with ageing, when a person gets dementia, friends and extended family often fall away. Some reasons are that friends don't know what to expect or how to interact with the person with dementia, they have stopped finding the relationship enjoyable or meaningful, they find the person with dementia difficult to deal with, and being with the person with dementia makes them confront their own mortality. Other reasons are that the carer declines invitations and avoids social situations to protect the person with dementia from being embarrassed or from losing face, or because they are worried that the person with dementia may behave inappropriately or spoil the social event for others. Other reasons are that the person with dementia tries to avoid social situations where they may make mistakes or their memory or other difficulties may be 'discovered', or that they seem to lose interest in organizing or making an effort to attend social functions.

Whatever the reason, losing their social circle is a big loss for the person with dementia, and often this loss is shared by the family carer, particularly the spouse. People with dementia value friendships and see friendships as important and as a close, nurturing, sharing relationship, in the same way people without dementia view friendships. But people with dementia, particularly in later stages of the disease, find it difficult to make new friends that meet this definition because of their difficulties in storing memories about new people. This makes keeping old friends especially important for people with dementia.

Many people with dementia and their family carers will not have the energy to keep as socially active as they were before the onset of the disease. They may also not want to maintain as large a social network.

TELLING FRIENDS AND FAMILY ABOUT A DIAGNOSIS OF DEMENTIA

We can think about our social network as a series of concentric circles, like the rings of an onion, with ourselves in the centre. The circle immediately around us holds the people nearest and dearest to us; this may be a spouse and/or best friend or friends. The circle around that holds good friends you can talk to about personal things and call on in times of need; there might be five to ten people in this second circle. The third circle holds more remote friends with whom you may spend social time but not necessarily confide in, and there could be five to 50 people in this circle. The outermost circle contains acquaintances whose names you might know but with whom you don't spend meaningful social time. Friends will drift in and out of circles over time.

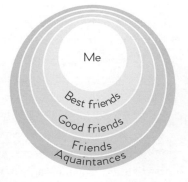

People with dementia and their carers usually tell the people in the inner circles of friendship first about the diagnosis of dementia. Some carers then tell everyone in the social network, whereas others don't spread the news as widely.

Sharing the diagnosis may be difficult for some people with dementia and their carers, especially for private people. However, telling others about the diagnosis of dementia makes it easier to keep friendships. Being honest means that you don't have to cover up memory difficulties or unusual behaviour. Once friends know, many will make allowances, making a special effort to be accommodating to routines and what might work better for the person with dementia and their carer. They are also more understanding that the person with dementia may be less able to reciprocate in the friendship than they used to. Telling others does involve the risk that they will stop being friends, but if this is the case they may have stopped being friends when they noticed the person with dementia's symptoms irrespective of whether the diagnosis was shared or not.

If you've talked about the diagnosis, this opens the door to having a conversation about the symptoms of the person with dementia, and discussion about how he could be treated. It is important to have these conversations with family as well. Share with your friends and family the specific difficulties with memory or thinking that the person has (the checklist in Chapter 1 will help you) and any behaviours that are unusual for that person. Specific information about symptoms rather than generic descriptions of dementia are more helpful. You may think that these difficulties are obvious, but their extent might not be as apparent to others who don't see them every day. Remind your friends and family also that in spite of the symptoms, the person with dementia is still the same person they were and continues to enjoy the company of others (if this is true).

Explain that if the person with dementia is in a group they might not want to be the focus of attention, preferring instead to sit and take in the scene around them. Ask relatives to take time to give the person one-on-one attention, even at group gatherings. Ask them to share an experience that they have had and then to listen to the person.

It is never too late to have this conversation with friends. True friends will understand if you phone them after several years and apologize for losing touch and explain the reasons why.

ASKING FAMILY TO BE MORE INVOLVED

Some families of people with dementia find that the illness brings them closer emotionally or in more frequent contact. However, there may be a family member who the rest of the family feels is not pulling their weight in terms of contributing to the person with dementia's life and care. This family member might not know their help is needed; or being with the person with dementia could make them feel uncomfortable. They might not see it as their responsibility to help or they may have circumstances that make it more difficult to contribute to the care of the person with dementia. In order for the situation to change, someone will need to let the person know that their help is needed. Sometimes this conversation is easy. In other instances, because of the family history or the person's personality, or a whole combination of different factors, this conversation can be more difficult. However, if we avoid having the conversation the situation will probably not change!

In situations where I am going to have a conversation that I anticipate will be difficult, I find it best to get mentally and emotionally prepared. The strategies suggested below may be helpful when having a difficult conversation with a family member, and are useful in any situations where there may potentially be two viewpoints and conflict, whether at work or at home. These are techniques that psychologists and other health professionals teach as part of negotiation skills and conflict management.

1. I figure out what the best-case outcome is, and also what a reasonable, though not ideal, outcome is. If I can't get everything I want, I ask myself what would I be prepared to settle for? Thinking this way helps me go into the conversation prepared to negotiate rather than fighting to win.

2. I figure out a logical argument to present about what I would like to happen and why. In the case of a person with dementia, you might say something like: 'I would like you to visit Mum more often because she sees so few people these days and I think she is lonely.' I also try to anticipate counter-arguments that the person could present and work out measured responses to these.

3. I practise in my head the things I want to say, such as 'I' statements including 'I think ...' and 'I feel ...'. However, I generally try to avoid 'I want ...'. When I am talking about the other person's behaviour, instead of interpreting their behaviour as a fact (e.g. 'You are not taking responsibility for our mother's care' or 'You are not pulling your weight') I state it as my feelings in response to their behaviour: 'I feel really exhausted at doing so much for Mum, I feel like it would be helpful if you could do more' or 'I'm worried about not making the right decisions about Mum's care; it makes me feel solely responsible when you're not really involved' or 'I think you're

avoiding visiting Mum and Dad, but I'm not sure why.' Using 'I' statements softens what you're saying and also gives the person the ability to give their own perspective.

4. During the discussion, I try to listen to the other person's perspective and acknowledge this and their feelings. I try to control my own feelings and be reasonable. I try to understand why they are behaving the way they are because this will help me find a solution that suits us both. I try to see shades of grey rather than black or white sides of the discussion.

5. I am assertive but not aggressive in trying to negotiate an outcome.

Case study

ANTONIO

Sofia wants her brother, Antonio Jr, to be more involved in Antonio's care. She wants him to visit during the week every week, rather than just arriving at Sunday family lunch, eating and leaving. She also wants her brother to be involved in making decisions about Antonio's future care and to be more appreciative of Maria and the caring she does. That's her best-case scenario. An improvement would be if he visits during the week every fortnight, and is involved in discussions about care. A very mild improvement would be if he was just more supportive of Maria and more involved in discussions about care. Sofia telephones Antonio Jr.

Sofia: 'I'm calling to talk to you about Mamma and Papa.'

Antonio Jr:'Yes?'

Sofia: 'I'm worried that Papa isn't doing much anymore and that he will get worse if he doesn't keep using his brain.'

Antonio Jr: 'I don't think he is so bad, he still can do a lot for himself.'

Sofia: 'Yes, he can, but he doesn't. He spends a lot of time just sitting around. He hardly ever goes out anymore, and he's stopped having his evening walks.'

Antonio Jr: 'I didn't realize that, I hadn't really noticed much change in him.'

Sofia: (thinking to herself *You don't spend enough time with them to notice anything!*) 'I think that it would be good for Papa if we all made an effort to visit him more often. I'm now visiting twice during the week. Do you think you could drop by after work one day a week? You could discuss the news with Papa maybe, or maybe read some of *La Fammia* newspaper to him. I'm sure you could stay for dinner too.'

Antonio Jr: 'I don't know ... I'm very busy ...'

Sofia: 'Please, Antonio. Mamma and Papa need a little help now that they are older.'

Antonio Jr: 'They seem to be doing fine to me.'

Sofia: 'Yes, and we want to keep it that way. That's

why we should visit more often. How about
you try it for a month and see how you go?'

Antonio Jr: (hesitantly) 'All right ...'

Sofia: 'If you are visiting more, then you will know
more about what is going on with them. I'd
like that, then you can be more involved in
thinking and planning for Papa's care.'

Antonio Jr: 'What decisions are there to make?'

Sofia: 'Well, none now, but we just have to start
thinking about what we will do if he gets
worse. For instance, should we put his name
on a nursing-home waiting list?'

Antonio Jr: 'He's not going to go into a nursing home,
he's not that bad!'

Sofia: 'I'm not saying he's going into a nursing
home. It's just something we need to
discuss in the future.'

[In the above example, Sofia explained why she wanted
Antonio Jr to visit more frequently. She used 'I' statements
and was careful not to be critical of his behaviour. She
stated her opinions as opinions rather than facts.

SOCIALIZING WITH FRIENDS AND EXTENDED FAMILY

Having friends and extended family visit, going to their houses or going out together are normal parts of most of our lives. Friends of people with dementia often run out of things to say and find the conversation going round and round or petering into silence, which can be uncomfortable. Make some suggestions to close friends about activities they can do with people with dementia. Small outings and activities may be more successful than conversations. Including a person with dementia in a group where they can listen and watch even though they don't participate actively can also be meaningful to that person.

Sometimes the family occasions that people with dementia attend are large, long family get-togethers. They often enjoy being part of these large gatherings, however the noise and number of people mean that they find it hard to follow conversations and might not be able to connect with individual people. Making family members aware of the need to spend one-on-one time with the person with dementia during the gathering can help. Consider organizing smaller gatherings of just three or four people, which will make it easier for the person with dementia to engage and continue their individual relationships with important people.

Case study

RUTH

Julie and Hannah are increasingly concerned that Ruth does not seem to be on friendly terms with any of the other residents in the unit. The other residents are understandably annoyed by some of Ruth's behaviours, namely going into their rooms and removing their belongings, constantly pacing around and not sharing the dolls. Ruth gets agitated when other residents are verbally critical of or show negative body language towards her. Hannah decides to call Helena, Ruth's friend who argued with Julie when they were deciding to admit Ruth to the nursing home — Helena believed that Julie and Hannah should have tried to care for Ruth at home. Helena also complained that the home was very difficult for her to visit because she no longer drove a car.

Hannah: 'I'm calling to talk about Mum.'

Helena: 'How is she?'

Hannah: 'Physically she is fine. But I don't think she is doing so well in Lilli Pilli Gardens. She hasn't settled in well, she hasn't made any friends. And while the staff are all very nice, I don't think they have warmed to her. They have their favourites and she is not a favourite.'

Helena: 'I told you that I was worried about what putting her in one of those places would do to her. So, what are you going to do?'

Hannah: 'Julie and I are worried that they are going to throw her out of that unit, because they are always telling us how anxious she is and how much attention she needs. They tell us all the things that she has done wrong to other residents, and how she won't participate in activities. They have put her on an anti-psychotic drug to calm her down, but I don't think it has worked except to make her more dopey. I feel like she is being treated like a naughty child, but I don't think she is purposefully doing anything wrong.'

Helena: 'Are the staff not well trained there, and have they got enough?'

Hannah: 'The staff seem to be always busy doing something with someone. They do have group activities there, cooking and craft, but Mum doesn't show any interest in them. They go on a bus trip once a week but they won't take her because they say she is a flight risk. We think she needs one-on-one attention from staff, but they don't have the staff to do this. But it is meant to be a very good facility, and all the other families seem to be happy with it. When I talk with the other families they don't seem to be having the troubles we have.'

Helena: 'How does your mum feel about it?'

Hannah: 'Well, she doesn't really like being there. She always asks to go home and hates it when we leave, which is really hard. But we can't look after her safely at home anymore.'

Helena: 'I'm sure your mum wants to go home. It must be horrible living with strangers.'

Hannah: 'That's the reason I'm calling. Julie and I are trying to see if we can get Mum a visitor every day of the week. We both go twice a week, and we're going to see if Raymond and Scott can drop in after work every fortnight. That leaves two more days. I know it is a little way for you, but I'm wondering if you would mind visiting her. I'm sure she would love to see you.'

Helena: 'Oh ...'

Hannah: 'I think Mum is really lonely. She doesn't seem to have any friends and she seems to annoy the other residents. She was such a caring person, I don't really understand why she doesn't get on with them. I think she needs friends to remind her of who she is. We're going as often as we can. Can you help please ... for Mum?'

Helena: 'I would like to ... but ... as you know it is very far for me and I don't drive anymore.'

Hannah: 'I know it is far, but she would so love to see you. Can we find some way of getting you there? How about if we pay for a taxi for you?'

Helena: 'Are you sure? It will be quite expensive.'

Hannah: 'The cost isn't important, the main thing is that Mum gets a visit from you.'

Helena: 'Okay.'

Hannah: 'Wonderful, thank you! She will be so happy to see you.'

Helena: 'What day would you like me to go?'

Hannah: 'Can you go on Friday every week? That is

the day they go on a bus trip without Mum and she seems really sad to be left out.'

Helena: 'It may be too much to go every week, maybe every two weeks? I can do most Fridays but on the first Friday of the month I meet our old nurses group for lunch.'

Hannah: 'I forgot about that group. You've been meeting for so long ... Could the group sometimes visit Mum for lunch, or before or after lunch? There is a little café near the unit.'

Helena: 'Maybe ... Darlena and Margaret drive, so we could all go together every few months and maybe eat afterwards. We always like trying somewhere different to eat and there are some nice cafés in that area.'

Hannah: 'That would be really good for Mum to see them all again.'

Helena: 'I will talk with them at our next lunch next week. We'll give it a try and see how it goes.'

Hannah: 'When you visit Mum, she likes to go for a walk round the garden, or to have a coffee at the café. She's still quite talkative though she doesn't always make sense. Sometimes she is quite lucid.'

Helena: 'I'm sure we'll be all right.'

Hannah: 'Thanks so much, Helena.'

Helena: 'Thanks for calling me, Hannah. I have been wondering how Ruth was going, but it's been hard for me to visit.'

Hannah: 'I'll give you my number, please give me a call if you're not coming or if you want to talk about her.'

Ruth really enjoyed Helena's visits. She reacted to her in the same way as when Julie and Hannah visit. Ruth was also very engaged when the lunch group visited her — she didn't seem to recognize all the group members but sat and listened to the conversation, and nodded and laughed appropriately. She wanted to go with them when they left. One member of the group, Darlena, lived in the local area and also started to visit Ruth when she was made aware of the situation.

The above example shows how friends can be asked for help in the social care of a person with dementia. Hannah had to put behind her a family quarrel to ask Helena for help. She gave a rationale for wanting Helena to visit, explaining about Ruth's mood and behaviour. She was also clear about what their family was doing and what help they wanted. Sometimes practical barriers have to be worked through. Hannah also was open to negotiating days and frequencies. Suggesting a trial group visit gave them the ability to try it before committing. Visitors don't know what to expect during the first visit, so suggesting a trial lets them try a visit before committing themselves regularly.

Case study

BRIAN

Gary and June have had little interaction with John, Brian's previous business partner, although they are aware through staff comments that John visits regularly. After hearing from staff that John hasn't visited for a while, Gary decides to contact him. Gary talks to John by phone.

Gary: 'Hello, John, this is Gary, Brian's nephew.'

John: 'Oh ... hello, Gary. What can I do for you?'

Gary: 'I'm ringing to check that you are okay. The staff at Uncle Brian's nursing home said you hadn't been to visit him for a while.'

John: 'Oh ... umm ... I've been away for a month ... on holiday.'

Gary: 'I'm glad you are okay. While I've got you on the phone, have you got a few minutes to talk about Uncle Brian?'

John: 'Yes, yes of course.'

Gary: 'We're finding it really difficult visiting Uncle Brian. Sometimes he gets angry at me, and sometimes we aren't sure if he recognizes us. June had the good idea of taking photographs and this has made things a little better. At least we have something to talk to him about and sometimes he even makes sense to us.'

John. 'Yes, yes, it is difficult.'

Gary: 'I'm really concerned that we're not doing all we can for him and he is sad and lonely in there. But we don't know what else to do. What do you think? When you visit him does he seem lonely? The staff say that Uncle Brian is always happy to see you.'

John: 'Well ... to be honest he is always happy to see me but he hates it when I leave. He hangs on to my arm and cries and gets angry at me when I'm trying to go.'

Gary: 'At least he is pleased to see you. What do you talk about?'

John: 'Well ... I usually take the newspaper and read him a few stories. Brian listens, but I think he understands less and less now of what is in there ... To be honest I haven't been on holiday, I just haven't been to visit your uncle because it's so difficult being with him.'

Gary: 'I see. It's not just us having the problem of not knowing what to do with him. Well, it's helped us taking Uncle Brian things from his past like photographs. Maybe you could try that.'

John: 'What could I take?'

Gary: 'How about some old catalogues from the business, or some old books? Or how about some machine components?'

John: 'That's a good idea. I may try those.'

Gary:	At least it gives you something else to talk about.'

Gary and John talk a little more about ideas for things to take to discuss with Brian.

John:	'I'm glad you called. It's given me a few ideas, and now at least I know when you visit and what you do with him.'
Gary:	'How about we leave a book in Uncle Brian's room that we both write in when we visit. A communication book. Then you can tell us what has worked, and if you really do go on holiday then we'll know.'
John:	'All right. That's a good idea.'

Gary and June place an exercise book in the top drawer of Brian's dresser to be a communication book between themselves and John. They write short notes about each visit. Angie, the staff member who takes the most interest in Brian, also writes in it sometimes, most often when she wants to tell Gary and June about something that Brian needs. Angie later reports that reading the little notes helps her understand Brian better and gives her things to chat to him about.

John starts to bring his toolbox, and nuts and bolts and other items relating to machinery on his visits. Each visit he does an activity and encourages Brian to help him and participate. He might clean and organize his toolbox, sort through the nuts and bolts jars and rearrange them, dismantle a small piece of machinery. If he can't think of a new activity he repeats one of the previous activities. With permission, he also works with Brian's help in the garden, pruning or weeding or sweeping together. One week they oil some of the doors in the unit because Angie had complained that they were squeaky. John finds it much more natural to relate in this way with Brian, and his visits are now sometimes much longer than they had been previously. Brian continues to be distressed when John leaves, so John has learnt to time his departure with mealtimes, when Brian can be partially distracted with lunch or afternoon tea.

The above example shows how different carers sharing their experiences can help generate ideas for interactions for people with dementia. John felt guilty about not visiting Brian yet was frustrated and exhausted when he did visit. Finding some strategies made the visits (though not the exits) more enjoyable for John and more engaging and stimulating for Brian. This also shows how communication between family, friends and professional staff can improve and give cohesion to the activities provided for persons with dementia.

TEENAGERS AND CHILDREN

Talk with teenagers and children at an appropriate level about the memory and thinking difficulties of the person with dementia and how this may affect their behaviour. There are books for younger children that may start the discussion about symptoms of dementia. I like *Wilfred Gordon McDonald Partridge* by Mem Fox and *The Memory Box* by Mary Bahr; there are many others.

Give the person with dementia and children things that they

can do together one on one. If the person with dementia can read, get them to read a book, or give them a toy that they can still manage and get them to help the child (e.g. reading, writing, craft, simple puzzles), sing a song together, draw pictures together.

Encourage children to 'show and tell' their experiences and things they are interested in (toys, books, fashion magazines, car models, gadgets) with the person with dementia. Get them to ask the person with dementia about their childhood. Encourage them to ask for advice and help, if the person with dementia is able to provide this. Older children and teenagers may be interested in putting together a photograph book of the person's life, or writing up or making a video about the family history. This joint project could be for a special occasion such as a birthday or family reunion.

If the interactions between the person with dementia and younger people can be scheduled regularly (once a fortnight or a month), the children can prepare for the visits and plan things to tell them. Telephone conversations between people with dementia and children don't work very well, but video conferencing may be more successful and could be tried for families that live far apart. Teenagers can be reluctant to visit (they are reluctant to do many things!), however they should be encouraged as part of their family and social obligations, and out of love for the older family member. Try to find an activity that the teenager can lead for the person with dementia.

Intergenerational programs, in which older people and younger people are encouraged to interact, have been shown to benefit both the older person and the younger person. These are usually built around an activity that the older person and younger person do together. The older person with dementia usually works with between one and three youngsters on an activity. Younger people often find older people interesting, enjoy their 'oldness' and life experience and appreciate that the older person has time for them. They seem to quite easily accept the older person as they are. Older people enjoy being experts and are energized by the enthusiasm and exuberance of youth. Examples of intergenerational programs include older people with dementia teaching or participating in Montessori activities with preschoolers, university students facilitating art experiences for people with dementia, and primary-school children and nursing-home residents singing together in a choir.

Case study

ANTONIO

Sofia has asked Tony, her son who is ten, to spend some time with his grandfather, Antonio. Tony complains that Antonio doesn't understand him when he speaks English, and he doesn't like speaking Italian. Sofia encourages Tony to spend a little time talking with his grandfather and suggests that his Italian might improve with practice. Sofia also talks about Antonio's memory difficulties and how this has made him lose touch with his friends, and how it is important for the family to keep his mind active so that his dementia does not get worse.

Tony: 'Ciao, Nonno.'

Antonio: 'Come stai, Tony?'

Tony: 'I'm well, Nonno. How are you?'

Antonio: 'Bene, bene.' (Tony looks at Sofia)

Sofia: 'Papa, Tony has been doing well in his football team.'

Antonio: 'Good, good. What position do you play?'

Tony: 'Well, I like to play striker, but sometimes I have to be a defender.'

Antonio: 'I played striker too.'

Tony: 'You did?'

Antonio: 'Yes, like Luigi Rivera.'

Tony: 'Were you good?'

Antonio: 'So so.'

Tony: 'My favourite soccer player is Tim Cahill.'

Antonio: 'Tim?'

Tony: 'You don't know him? He's a Socceroo.'

Antonio: 'You should support the Azzuri.'

Tony: 'But we live here in Australia, we need to support the Australian team.'

Antonio: 'Australia? You are Italian. You should support the Azzuri.'

Tony: 'I don't know much about them.'

Antonio: 'I will take you to Brunswick to a game.'

Tony: 'But the Azzuri don't play in Brunswick.'

Antonio: 'Yes they do, I have seen them play many times.'

Sofia: 'Tony, don't argue with Nonno, please.'

Tony: 'But Mum ...'

Sofia: 'Tony ...'

Sofia gets Tony to look up Brunswick Juventus on the internet. Tony discovers that some famous Socceroo players played for the club. He prints out some pictures of these players and takes them on his next visit to his grandfather.

Tony: 'Nonno, look at these players. This is Paul Wade, Charlie Egan. They played for your club, Juventus.'

Antonio: 'Paul Wade.'

Tony: 'Do you know him?'

Antonio: 'Of course, of course. He played for us.'

Tony: 'Did you ever meet him?'

Antonio: 'Of course.'

Tony: 'Wow! What was he like?'

Antonio: 'A good player.'

Tony: 'What other players did you know?'

Antonio: 'Our best team was in that year that we didn't win. But we should have won.'

Tony: 'I've been watching ...' (goes into a story about games that he has been watching)

Antonio: 'Good, good.'

Tony: 'Would you like to watch a game with me? Maybe we can watch one now.'

Antonio: 'Yes, sure.'

Tony and Antonio then watch highlights of a soccer game together. Antonio zones out for part of it, but Tony chats to him excitedly about the players and score, and Antonio comments briefly on plays and tactics. Sofia comments to Maria afterwards that it was great for Tony to still be able to relate to Antonio, and Maria says that even though Antonio struggled to follow the whole game he participated and commentated and was very tired when Tony left.

The next week Tony brings a soccer board game. Antonio agrees to play but doesn't follow Tony's rather contorted explanation of the rules. Nonetheless, they cooperate to play the game happily.

This example demonstrates how children will accommodate the shortcomings of a person with dementia and figure out how to interact in a way that suits their own interests. Having a common interest helped Tony and Antonio connect. An adult may need to help facilitate the development of the relationship between child and person with dementia by helping the child understand the background and behaviour of the person with dementia.

DON'T EXPECT TO KEEP ALL FRIENDSHIPS

Sometimes friends have differing opinions about how to treat or care for the person with dementia. Sometimes you can agree to disagree; in other instances it is extremely difficult to stay friends when there is strong disagreement.

There may be some friends who, through their interactions with the person with dementia — such as by talking over him or as if he is not there, or talking down to him — make that person feel inadequate. It is worthwhile considering the value of the friendship to the person with dementia and to the carer if it is not a positive relationship. It is probably not realistic to expect to keep all, or even most, of the person with dementia's and family carer's friends.

PRACTICAL TIPS

There is a lot of stigma (negative attitudes and beliefs) around dementia. People in the community may feel uncomfortable and awkward around someone with dementia because they no longer know how to act around them.

For friends who seem to be finding it difficult to know how to interact with the person with dementia (and even for those who don't), it might help to write down (in collaboration with the person with dementia if she is able) some information about the difficulties she is having with memory or thinking or day-to-day tasks, as well as what friends can do to help. Writing it down saves explaining it multiple times to different people, and gives them something they can read and think about in their own time. It might also help them be more comfortable around the person with dementia.

Here is an example of what you could write down:

I have a diagnosis of dementia. Please continue to treat me as your friend. If I behave in an unusual way, it may be because of trouble I'm having with my memory. Here are some of my difficulties and how you can help:

My difficulties	How you can help me
I forget things I have done recently, such as in the past day/week/month	Don't ask me too many questions about recent events
I forget the names of people I am familiar with	Remind me of your name if I seem to have forgotten it
I sometimes forget what I am saying in the middle of a conversation	Remind me of what I was talking about if I seem to lose track
I sometimes get flustered or overreact about a situation that I think I can't manage	Help me to calm down, find me somewhere quiet to sit and a cup of coffee

8

GOING OUT

The purpose of outings is to leave the home and go somewhere to see, hear, smell, taste or do something different. A change of environment activates different brain areas than those used in our home routines, and stimulates different thoughts.

Some people with dementia are reluctant to leave home, their place of safety. Some want to know that they are with someone they can trust to keep them safe when they are out. If the person with dementia is reluctant to go out, try to figure out why. What are they worried about when they go out? Is it something that might happen to them while they are out? Or are they worried about what will happen to the home while they are away? If you can figure out what it is, then you can try to address their concerns.

Agoraphobia is a mental health disorder where the person has a fear of being in an inescapable situation or where help would be unavailable and is often associated with a fear of leaving home. Agoraphobia is rare, occurring in less than 1 per cent of older adults. If the person you are caring for has agoraphobia, then it would be extremely difficult for you to persuade them to go out for recreational reasons. Psychological therapies tend to be successful in treating agoraphobia, so if you suspect that the person has agoraphobia or another mental health disorder, seek diagnosis and treatment.

A CHANCE FOR A 'NORMAL' LIFE AND RELATIONSHIP

After developing dementia, the lives of people with dementia and their carers change significantly. Their relationship changes significantly too, as one person becomes much more dependent on the other both around the house and in life more generally. The dependent person loses control and power in the relationship. Spouse carers say that sometimes it is important to feel normal and be a 'couple' again. Family carers say how important it is to sometimes just spend time with their relative with dementia without being specifically in the caring role. Outings provide an opportunity for the person with dementia and their carer to interact in a more normal and equal way.

SHORT OUTINGS

Here are some suggestions for short outings around your local area. You may be able to do these every day by walking and driving:

- to the shops
- around a park
- a walk along the beach or river
- to the playground to watch the children play
- to the football pitch to watch an amateur game
- to a café for a tea of coffee
- to look at progress on a construction site

- to feed the birds
- to have an ice-cream or hot chips
- to have a picnic
- to a religious service.

LONGER OUTINGS

Longer outings give us something to look forward to, a reason to get dressed in our good clothing and something interesting to talk about later. Longer outings often take a little more organization, and you might be able to do these once a week or once every few weeks. Here are suggestions for longer outings:

- go out for a nice meal
- go to visit a friend or relative
- go to a concert, museum, art gallery
- go into 'town'
- go to a market.

If you're planning a longer outing, try to avoid situations where there will be a lot of noise and/or crowds, because people with dementia find it difficult to concentrate in these situations and can feel stressed. If you want to go to a concert, a short intimate lunchtime concert may be better for the person with dementia than a long evening concert with a big audience. If you are going to a concert, if possible sit near the front on the side so you can leave early if necessary, and so that the person with dementia doesn't have to spend energy filtering out the rest of the crowd in front of them and can concentrate on the show. Similarly, avoid going to galleries, museums and markets when they are crowded such as in the middle of the day on weekends. Before you go to a gallery or museum, plan the exhibits you want to see and don't make the visit too long.

If you do go on a longer, bigger outing, take photographs so that you can talk about what you've done afterwards. You can plug the memory card from your digital camera directly into a digital photo frame to help the person with dementia experience the pleasure of the outing again.

During outings, conversations tend to be in the moment. Help the person with dementia observe their surroundings and talk about the people and things around them that they can see, hear, feel and smell. Give the person time to look around them and reflect on what they see and hear. The outing could bring up old memories that the person with dementia wants to reminisce about.

DEMENTIA-SPECIFIC OUTINGS

There are services that provide opportunities for people with dementia and their carers to have social or cultural experiences in dementia-friendly environments. Your local Alzheimer's association is a good place to start finding out what services are available in your local area (see also 'Further resources', p. 230). Here are some services that I have heard wonderful stories about:

Dementia cafés

These cafés are organized gatherings where people with dementia and their family carers can 'drop in' and enjoy time together with some refreshments and entertainment. The environment is supportive, as all the people who attend are in a similar situation, and there are professional staff available who coordinate activities and provide information and advice.

Dementia dinner and dances and dementia restaurants

These provide opportunities for people with dementia and their family carer to go out for a social occasion. The restaurants often offer a three-course meal in an environment that is not too noisy and with supportive staff. The dinner and dances offer a meal and organized free dancing with music from the appropriate era.

Art gallery and museum tours for people with dementia

Art gallery tours were conceptualized and started by the ARTZ organization in the United States. The program was then piloted in Australia at the National Gallery of Australia. Evaluation found that people with dementia enjoyed and were engaged in the program, and talked and participated much more than their carers expected. Family carers also enjoyed the program. There were no measurable improvements in mood, behaviour or quality of life of the people with dementia overall, but the evaluation team still believed that the program had value and the benefits were encapsulated in the comment by one participant: 'You do it for the moment.'

Given its success, the art gallery and museum program has been made available in several urban and regional art galleries around Australia (ask your institution if they run a program for people with dementia). The program involves selecting artworks that would be interesting and engaging for people with dementia and training museum educators on leading tours for people with dementia. The tours are usually open to people with dementia living at home or in nursing homes, and their carers.

Choirs for people with dementia

There is good evidence that many people with dementia enjoy participating in a choir and are very proud to perform to an audience! There is also some evidence that participating in choirs improves the mood and wellbeing of people with dementia. Family carers are usually welcome to also participate in these choirs and some nursing homes have facility choirs. I have also seen bell choirs for people with dementia, where instead of singing, each person rings one or two bells under the direction of a conductor.

Men's Sheds for people with dementia

The Australian Men's Shed Association is a community-based organization that provides an opportunity for men, including those with dementia, to have a 'male' space in which to spend time and complete meaningful projects and activities. There may be organized projects to which the men contribute such as simple assembly, sanding or painting. There are also tools to be cleaned and sorted and stored. The concept has now spread to New Zealand, Ireland and the United Kingdom.

OTHER INTERNATIONAL PROGRAMS

The following programs show how activities can be modified for groups of people with dementia to enjoy. Check 'Further resources' (p. 230) for details on how to access programs in your area (note that, at the time of writing, these programs have not yet reached Australia but they may give you some inspiration).

Concerts and movies

In the United Kingdom there are occasionally concerts by choirs and orchestras specifically for people with dementia and their carers. The time of day, setting and program are created to be more suitable for people with dementia.

ARTZ in the United States run a program called 'Meet me at the movies' where key scenes from old movies are shown in a cinema, followed by discussion and reminiscence. The clips are selected based on interviews with people with dementia to be resonant with them, and trained staff support the participants through the activity. This concept has been adopted by professional care staff who put on a 'movie day', and family carers could also do this at home. It would also be a nice idea for an intergenerational activity.

Holidays

There are UK companies that specialize in holidays for people with dementia and their families (as far as I know there are none in Australia but you might like to investigate whether anyone offers this service in other countries). These companies offer accommodation, or guided tours and activities, with increased practical help and a supportive social environment as part of the service.

PRACTICAL CONSIDERATIONS

There are logistical considerations that you need to plan so that any outing can proceed as smoothly as possible. For instance, you don't want to have the person with dementia hungry and grumpy and not knowing where to get food, or needing to use the toilet and not knowing where the nearest facilities are. Some things to consider include:

- What and when will we eat?
- Where are the nearest toilets? National and local area maps of public toilets are often available; check 'Further resources' (p. 230) for more information.
- How will we get there? How long will it take? Is there parking if we need it?
- What will the weather be like?
- Will many other people be there, and how might that impact our outing?
- Are there any places where we may have to wait in line, and can we minimize this by pre-paying for tickets or making a booking?

Case study

BRIAN

Gary and June decide to try to take Brian out for a drive to see the neighbourhood where he grew up. They discuss the outing in detail as he has not left the nursing home for over a year. They decide they can manage an outing where he stays in the car, and they pack food in case he is hungry. They wait for a day where he is not grumpy and is relatively agreeable. To introduce the idea of the outing they show him some photos of himself at his old home.

Gary: 'Uncle Brian, would you like to go and see your old house?' (Brian looks at the photograph.)

Gary: 'Uncle Brian, would you like to go to the place where this photo was taken?'

Brian: 'Yes.'

Brian is uncharacteristically cooperative in going to the toilet, having his shoes put on and getting into the car. June chats to him about the weather and things around them. Brian doesn't talk but he seems to be listening and nods. Brian looks around during the drive and seems particularly interested when they drive past paddocks with sheep in them. Gary and June decide to pull over so that Brian can have a better look at a paddock with several ewes and lambs. Brian tries to open the door, so they cautiously help him out of the car and over to the fence to look at the sheep. He doesn't stand still to look at the sheep, though; he walks slowly and determinedly along the fence.

'Uncle Brian,' says Gary, 'where are you going? Look, the sheep are here. Look, sheep.' Gary tries to take Brian's arm to bring him back to the fence and the car. But Brian shakes him off and keeps going.

'Uncle Brian, come on,' he says.

Brian walks round the corner of the fence and keeps going until he comes to a gate. He tries to open this but is unable to figure out the mechanism.

'Uncle Brian, it's locked,' Gary tells him. 'Come back to the car. We're going to see your old house.'

Brian keeps shaking the gate to try to open it and won't be dissuaded. Gary and June decide that since Brian is so determined, they will let Brian trespass on the property and they open the gate for him. He makes directly for the sheep; Gary and June follow him, ready to intervene if anything dangerous happens. Brian stops about 4 metres from the sheep. They turn to look at him but don't move away. Brian then moves slowly towards them.

'Uncle Brian, what are you doing?' asks Gary. 'Uncle Brian, these aren't our sheep.' Brian stops.

'Uncle Brian, we don't need to look after these sheep. They aren't our sheep.' Brian keeps looking at the sheep. He then turns around and starts walking towards the fence.

'The gate is this way,' says Gary. Brian lets Gary lead him towards the gate and gets into the car. He falls asleep in the car and they take him back to the nursing home.

Gary and June were happy to see Brian actively involved in his environment during the outing. The nursing-home staff report that he ate well that evening. Once a month from then on, Gary and June took Brian for 'drives', which he usually seemed to enjoy. This continued even as his dementia deteriorated, even though it was quite an effort to get him into the car. They stopped when they could no longer get him into the car.

The above example shows Gary and June following Brian's lead and interest while at the same time trying to keep him safe. It also shows them trying to interpret the intent of his behaviour, and when it was potentially going to be dangerous, intervening in a manner consistent with what they believed his thoughts were (to catch or interact in some way with the sheep). For June and Gary, the outings made their visits more worthwhile and meaningful and enjoyable.

BEING OUT IN PUBLIC AND STIGMA

Some carers are concerned about how the person with dementia might be perceived or treated when out in public, particularly if they have unusual behaviours. There have been increasing and ongoing awareness campaigns about what the symptoms of dementia are, and how to treat people who may be confused or behaving unusually. Governments and councils are also beginning to create age-friendly and dementia-friendly communities. The hope is that, by increasing awareness, the stigma experienced by persons with dementia and their carers will decrease.

When we do experience stigma of any sort, such as racism or sexism, sometimes we are so shocked or taken aback that we don't know how to react. We then find ourselves thinking afterwards of all the things we should or could have said or done. It helps carers to think ahead about what we could do or say if someone acts in a critical or derogatory way towards the person with dementia. Would you take the person with dementia out of the situation? Would you try to explain to the critical person that the person has dementia and has a bad memory, or has poor judgment, or has forgotten his social etiquette? Would you just smile and try to not worry about the comments? How about the reaction of the person with dementia — if she is upset about the comments would you downplay them, or say that the other person was being rude? As a carer how would you feel to be with the person with dementia when they don't behave according to social norms? Try to steel yourself to not be embarrassed no matter how the person with dementia (or other people) behaves; just because they don't behave according to social norms doesn't mean the person with dementia has no right to participate in community activities.

My view is that if you think others in your community (friends, neighbours, local shopkeepers) will be receptive you should tell them that the person in question has dementia — importantly, however, this must only be done with the permission of the person with dementia. I would also explain that she is still a person and should be treated with dignity and respect, even if she has a bad memory or behaves in unusual ways. Being open is one way of decreasing stigma in the community. Sharing this information may be the start of a deeper conversation about dementia. I've found that many people have some personal experience with a person with dementia and are understanding, sympathetic or empathetic when such a disclosure is made. Some people are also curious and want to ask questions, so be prepared to share a little about your experiences.

Case study

JOY

Bernie wants to take Joy on holiday. He grapples with this decision, given the importance of routine for people with dementia and the potential that she could find the holiday distressing or difficult. On the other hand, he feels that he'd like a change of scenery and that Joy might enjoy the holiday too. Bernie discusses the possibility of going on holiday with Joy, and she seems keen to go.

After some research, Bernie decides they will go on a cruise from Sydney to Tasmania. He does this to minimize air travel and because it will allow them to have the routine of the same hotel room for the whole trip. He selects a cruise company with a reputation for being good at looking after older travellers. He then contacts the company to see if it is possible to have a little additional support, such as the same table booked for each mealtime, and a state room with big windows that is close to the middle of the ship.

In preparation for the trip, Bernie makes a note of items that Joy seems to use often in their daily routine. He packs many of these for use during their trip. This includes their kitchen calendar, a large bedside clock, her make-up kit and a photograph of them that she has on her bedside table. Bernie decides it is safer to over-pack than not take an important item.

Bernie has many enjoyable discussions with Joy in anticipation of the trip, looking at photographs of the ship, its amenities and state rooms. They do some imagining of how they are going to live in the lap of luxury for seven days. Joy seems excited that they are going on the trip and near the departure date keeps asking how long until they go.

When they arrive at the ship, Bernie unpacks with Joy's help, hanging up Joy's clothes and putting out her toiletry items where they are visible on top of the vanity rather than placing them in a drawer. The toilet door is somewhat camouflaged by the panelling, so he gets a piece of paper, writes 'toilet' and sticks it on the door. They write Joy's name and room number on a card, and place both the key and card on a lanyard for Joy to wear around her neck. With Joy's agreement, they also talk to the ship's cruise director about Joy's dementia and ask that if staff find Joy alone, lost or disoriented, to walk her back her to her room and keep her company and page

Bernie. Joy says that she is confident she will be fine and that if she gets lost, she will just wait until Bernie comes to find her. For the first few days Joy sticks by Bernie's side very closely, but as they spend more time on the ship Joy's confidence grows.

On the first afternoon, Bernie and Joy spend time chatting to another older couple. The next day when they meet this couple again, Joy has forgotten them. This leads to a somewhat awkward conversation where the couple seem to think that Joy is being rude to them. Bernie struggles in deciding whether or not to explain to them that Joy has dementia. He decides to ask Joy's permission to tell them (without reminding her that they have met previously), with the explanation that they may be nice people to keep company with throughout the cruise. Joy agrees. Bernie then finds the opportunity to tell the other couple about Joy's memory difficulties while she is in the powder room. Disappointingly, Bernie finds that the couple do not seem to know how to react to his revelation, and are cool and seem to avoid them for the rest of the cruise. Luckily, Joy has forgotten them and doesn't realize she is being snubbed.

Otherwise the cruise is extremely enjoyable for Joy and Bernie. The cruise director and other staff seem to spend extra time talking with them and making them comfortable. The shorter day excursions they choose to do are well planned, and again staff are very supportive without being intrusive.

When they return home, aided by photos placed around the house, Joy talks enthusiastically about their trip for over a week before seeming to forget about it.

This example illustrates the planning and thought that went into a successful holiday. It also shows some of the social difficulties that may arise from being in a tour group.

PHYSICAL EXERCISE

Exercise is good for all of us. It is good for our physical health and mental health.

There is also a growing body of research suggesting that physical activity can improve memory and thinking for people with dementia. To date the studies have been small and not scientifically rigorous, and not all have produced benefits on mental abilities. It is not clear what type of exercise and how much is beneficial, but experts think that exercise with an aerobic component for a total of 150 minutes a week may improve memory and thinking in people with mild to moderate dementia. As most exercise programs studied have been run in groups, the social aspect may also be important. These exercise programs also seem to improve mood and depression in people with dementia.

Exercise does not have to be a chore or separate activity, it can be part of other activities such as transport, housework or recreation. The recommendation for physical activity for older adults is to do at least 30 minutes of moderately intense physical activity on most, preferably all, days. This should incorporate fitness, strength, balance and flexibility. A moderate level of activity noticeably increases your heart rate and breathing rate. You might sweat but you are still able to carry on a conversation. You can talk but you can't sing.

If you want to plan physical activities for people with dementia, then make them meaningful. If there is a sport the person previously enjoyed, then present a modification of that sport — for instance, golfers might enjoy mini golf or putting towards a target, or walking around a golf course. A netball player might enjoy catching and throwing a ball. Entertainment systems such as Wii offer another way to play 'sport'.

If the person did not previously play sport then make sure that exercise is fun and interactive. Many cognitively intact adults do not do physical activity even though it is good for them, so it is very unlikely that a person with dementia will do exercise just because it is good for them.

Here are some ideas for physical activities that can be made social or fun:

- walking in a group
- dancing to music
- throwing and catching a ball, small bean bag or soft toy — this can be with another person or into a vessel
- bouncing a ball
- rolling a ball towards a target (like bowling)
- hitting a ball against a wall
- kicking a ball (can be done sitting).

9

ACTIVITIES AROUND THE HOME

Activities around the home make up the rhythm of daily life. Getting bathed, dressed and groomed are events that happen from the beginning of our lives and form part of our daily routine, marking out mornings from afternoons, and afternoons from evenings. Housework, cooking and gardening are also part of most adult routines. Hobbies such as art and craft are also often part of our weekly lives.

When we go on holiday most of us enjoy the break from housework. Some of us even get a break from personal care by being bathed and groomed by others as part of spa or hairdressing treatments. I find that after a week at a resort, where almost everything is done for me, I get bored and I miss the privacy, control and satisfaction of doing many things for myself. I know some of you may disagree, and would be happy to have someone else do the domestics all the time!

Most of us think of housework and self-care as mentally easy, even though it may be physically demanding. This is because we've practised these skills so much that they are done based on our procedural memory. When someone who has not done a household task attempts it for the first time, it is not as easy as we take for granted. Children's early play is often based around household activities and they practise these skills repeatedly until they master them. We've all heard a story about someone (usually a man) who has never done laundry in his life, who suddenly has to wash his own clothes. He doesn't know how to operate the washing machine or how much powder to put in. When after some effort he successfully puts on a load, he dyes a white shirt pink or shrinks a woollen jumper.

When we use task analysis to break down the steps involved in an 'easy' task such as getting dressed, we realize how cognitively complex the task is, and how there is great potential for a person with dementia to run into difficulties:

1. Work out what the weather is currently like and what it might be like for the rest of the day. This judgment could be made by looking out the window, looking up the weather forecast or using general knowledge of the weather at that time of year — for instance there may be a broad temperature difference between early morning and noon which needs to be taken into consideration. Work out what activities will occur that day.

2. Based on the above, select clothes appropriate for current and potential weather and for planned activities, as well as matching aesthetically. Ensure that all required pieces of clothing are selected, including underwear and socks, and outerwear such as jacket and hat if needed.

3. Get dressed, putting the items on in the appropriate order. Each clothing item needs to be oriented the correct way before being put on, for instance, making

sure that it is not inside out or back to front. Some items may need to be put on in a specific order — for instance put a T-shirt on over the head before putting the arms into the sleeves. After putting on an item it may need to be adjusted on the body — for instance smoothing down sleeves under a jumper. Some clothing needs to be fastened appropriately with buttons, zips, buckles or ties.

4. Check in a mirror that the ensemble all looks okay, and if not, adjust as appropriate.

DO WITH RATHER THAN DO FOR

Many people with dementia give up personal self-care. Sometimes it is because they are unable to do some or all of the steps; for instance when getting dressed they may not be able to choose appropriate clothing. Sometimes it is because they can do the activity but they do not initiate it. Sometimes it is because well-meaning carers do these things for them.

Family carers often see doing housework and personal care as part of their caring role. Professional carers see it as part of their job. I agree, to some extent. But I think it is the family and professional carer's role to *help* the person with their personal care and housework, not do these tasks for them. By doing tasks for someone else we take away their choice and control, any sense of accomplishment or success in completing the task and any sense of self associated with the task. We're also taking away opportunities to exercise the body and mind, which incrementally may impact on their mental and physical function. Think how quickly you can get out of shape when you're sick at home in bed for a week; all the small things we do around the house contribute to keeping us in shape.

In residential care, there is an expectation from families and staff that they are paying the nursing home to look after the person, and this means that the nursing-home staff do things for the person in care. It takes a shift of mentality to think of nursing-home staff not as hotel staff but as life coaches whose job is to contribute therapeutically by helping the person with dementia to do as much as possible for themselves.

INVOLVING PEOPLE WITH DEMENTIA IN HOUSEWORK AND SELF-CARE

As far as is safe and practically possible, involve the person with dementia in housework and self-care activities. Choose activities that would be meaningful for them to be involved in. Meaningful household tasks are jobs that they might have previously done. To the person, the task might mean more than just completing a household chore; it might also mean that they have done something useful, contributed to the household and looked after their family.

The systematic way to modify activities to make them achievable for people with dementia is to subject each activity to task analysis. However, since this is time consuming you might not want to do this for every activity, so over the page are some ideas for modifications and support of household activities. Generally the person may have difficulty getting the different equipment needed and starting the activity; he may also have difficulty at points where another step needs to be initiated or a decision needs to be made. It will usually take longer to support a person doing a task than doing it for him. Doing a task together also usually involves much more interaction between the carer and the person with dementia, than if the carer just did the task alone.

Self-care

- Showering or bathing: Help the person choose and lay out things she will need such as clothes, towels and soap. Prompt or instruct at each step that she seems to be having difficulty with. Physically help when needed.
- Dressing: Help the person choose and lay out clothing in the order she will put the items on. Prompt or physically help with putting clothes on.
- Grooming: Encourage the person to comb or brush hair and wash her hands and face. You can 'touch up' her hair afterwards if needed. It may help to have the hair cut into a low-maintenance style.

Housework

Many of these tasks are sometimes done by a few people together, so it will feel more natural that there are two of you doing these tasks.

- Dusting or sweeping: Help him find the broom and pan or duster, and show him the dusty or dirty areas; he might also need to be shown how to collect and dispose of the dirt that has been collected.
- Laundry (hanging out, folding, sorting): Show him the work spaces for hanging or folding or sorting. If needed, give him only items he can manage in size and shape, for example small items such as handkerchiefs, socks and tea towels might be easier to manage.
- Setting the table: Help him locate the items that need to go on the table and remind him how the table should be set, for instance lay out one table setting for him to copy, and place mats to indicate where each setting should go.

- Cooking: Help him with the steps and order to prepare a simple meal such as a sandwich or toast and tea. Involve him in meal preparation by giving him tasks such as preparing and cutting up vegetables, stirring and mixing (e.g. batter, eggs) or kneading dough. He can also be involved in tasting and commenting on the food.
- Washing up: Prompt him to wash, rinse or dry dishes; set up a system for selecting the dirty dishes and stacking the clean dishes to make it as easy as possible.

Gardening

- Raking or sweeping: Help her find the rake or broom and show her areas that need raking or sweeping.
- Weeding or deadheading: Help her find the gloves and spade or secateurs, and show her where the weeds and dead flowers are.
- Planting (digging or filling pots with soil, planting, watering afterwards): Help her find the equipment she'll need (e.g. spade, seeds, watering can) and prompt or instruct as needed through the steps.
- Watering: Help her find and work the hose and tap, and show her the areas that need watering.

Hobbies

Generally, the person with dementia will need help in the planning component of a project. She may be able to choose what she wants to do, for instance she might want to knit a baby hat, but might need help choosing the pattern and size, amount and thickness of wool and appropriate needles. She might also need help with the order of activities, for instance deciding whether to paint the components of a footstool before assembling it or whether to assemble before painting.

Hobbies for men might involve assembly projects: building from a kit (furniture, model aircraft or cars or trains), painting something already assembled, or taking something apart then cleaning it and assembling it again. The person with dementia might need help with the assembly order.

Case study

ANTONIO

Maria asks Antonio to help her spring clean the pantry. Before starting, she gets ready cardboard boxes, a garbage bag, cleaning products and labels. The following conversations would have been carried out in Italian.

Maria: 'Antonio, I need your help.'

Antonio: 'What can I help with, *bella*?'

Maria: 'I need your help tidying the pantry.'

Antonio: 'I'm tired today ... it is nice sitting here.'

Maria: 'Please, Antonio. It is a lot of work and it will be faster if you help me.'

Antonio: 'Are you sure you need my help? I'm too old and slow to do things now.'

Maria: 'Of course I need your help. Four hands work faster than two. It would make me happy.'

Antonio: 'All right, I like making you happy.'

Maria: 'Thank you, my darling.'

Maria demonstrates with a few items how she wants to take everything out of the cupboard and put them in boxes then store them on or under the kitchen table. Antonio starts unpacking while Maria checks the expiry dates on each packet and throws away items that are old. After all the shelves have been unpacked, Maria demonstrates to Antonio how to spray and wipe the shelves. He does this while Maria follows with a clean cloth and water, wiping over them again. They do this companionably.

Antonio: 'Pasta from Italy is better than Australian pasta.'

Maria: 'Why do you think it is better?'

Antonio: 'The wheat is better. And the texture of the pasta is rougher. They use bronze machines to make it.'

Maria: 'I agree.'

A little while later:

Maria: 'This sugo is all past its date. I should throw it away.'

Antonio: 'It will be fine, we can smell it before we eat it. Sugo lasts a long time.'

Maria: 'We haven't made sugo in a while.'

Antonio: 'No, we have not.'

Maria: 'I'm not sure that I can remember how to make it.'

Antonio: 'Well, we need to buy tomatoes at the end of autumn when they are sweet and good. Then we need to crush them in the machine, and pass them through the cloth

to get rid of all the seeds and skins. Then
we need to fill our clean bottles and boil boil
boil.'

Maria: 'Yes, that is how we used to do it.'

Antonio: 'It would be good to make sugo this year.'

Maria: 'Yes, let's do that.'

The next day Maria labels the shelves and Antonio
restacks the cans and packets. Unprompted this time,
Antonio again tells the story about how to make sugo.

When they are finished packing the shelves, Antonio
admires their work with a smile on his face. 'We did a
good job,' he says. 'It is very tidy now.' He puts his arm
around his wife's shoulders affectionately.

This example shows how Maria gave supervision and clear
instructions about the task and made it easy for Antonio to
succeed. Providing boxes for Antonio to put the items from the
pantry in made the unpacking easier for him (he didn't have
to decide where to put them, and also each box could be put
away after it was filled, minimizing the clutter in the room).
It also showed how handling objects can sometimes stimulate
memories, and once they have been recalled they are easier to
access the next time. Maria felt closer and more connected to
Antonio because they were working together, as they used to do
in their convenience store, rather than seeing him as someone
who needs to be looked after.

CREATING ACTIVITIES BASED ON HOUSEHOLD TASKS

A person's level of dementia may deteriorate such that they would struggle to complete any household task, or the person with dementia might live in a nursing home where it is not possible to involve them in some household tasks. Some nursing homes are built to be homelike, with a working kitchen and laundry for residents to work and be involved in; however, in other homes residents do not have access to these facilities.

In these situations, we can create activities using household objects that may still hold meaning for the person because of their association with household activities, or because of their familiarity with the procedures. These activities involve manipulating, ordering and transforming objects in some way.

Here are some ideas for activities based on household objects. Treat these as starting ideas; you will come up with many others using items from around the home.

- Match, sort or sequence household items by category, shape, or colour — there are lots of items that can be sorted once you start looking for them such as socks, cutlery, tea towels, face washers, glasses, plates or hair rollers. Some things can also be arranged aesthetically such as arranging glasses in alternate colours, or flower arranging. Sequences could be from big to small or short to tall.
- Transfer objects from one container to another. This could be done by pouring (sand, water, beans, rice) or by transferring with fingers, spoons, scoops or tongs.
- Manipulate objects in other ways. For instance, peg clothes pegs to the edge of a basket, stretch rubber bands around a paper roll or cup, cut paper or card with

scissors or shears, chop fruit, thread beads or shoes, lace objects or shoes, wrap a present with paper and ribbon.

- Touch and interact with the objects sensorially. Some people with severe dementia may not have the manual dexterity or cognitive ability to complete the tasks above. They may enjoy touching and interacting with different objects, particularly ones they do not have access to in their usual environment. Giving them a bag of objects from your kitchen drawer, or the contents of a dressing-table drawer or a tool box can give them a variety of stimulating objects to interact with.

Case study

RUTH

Ruth refuses to participate in most of the activities offered in the nursing home. Kata reviews Ruth's life history to see if this will help her come up with ideas for activities that will engage her. She decides to see if Ruth would be interested in nursing-related activities. The two examples below show how manipulative activities can be tailored using simple objects available around most homes.

Kata: 'Hello, Ruth. It's Kata.'

Ruth: 'Hello.'

Kata: 'Ruth, I have a nursing job to do, will you help me?'

Ruth: 'Yes, anything for you, dear.'

Kata: 'I have this big bag of bandages, but they

	are a big mess. Can you help me roll them and put them in these baskets?'
Ruth:	'Yes.' (Ruth starts looking at the big pile of bandages for somewhere to start. Kata locates the end of a bandage and pulls it out.)
Kata:	'Here is the end of one.'
Ruth:	'Thank you.' (Ruth rolls up the bandage swiftly and dextrously. She looks for a way of fastening it.)
Kata:	'Oh, we don't have any clips to fasten them. Maybe you can just put it down in this basket for now.' (Kata points at where she wants Ruth to put the bandage, and then hands Ruth another bandage.)
Ruth:	'Some of these are dirty.'
Kata:	'Oh ... I didn't realize.'
Ruth:	'We should wash them all before we use them.'
Kata:	'Good idea.' (Ruth and Kata continue to roll bandages together until they are all done.)
Kata:	'Thank you for your help with these, Ruth.'
Ruth:	'Any time.'

Kata decides to try other nursing-related activities with Ruth. She brings her tweezers and cotton balls soaked in water in a stainless-steel medical tray, and a glass jar.

Kata:	'Hello, Ruth. It's Kata.'
Ruth:	'Hello.'
Kata:	'I've got these cotton balls here that are sterile, and I need to transfer them to this jar with these tweezers. It is important that we don't touch them with our fingers. Will you help me?'
Ruth:	'Okay, if I can.'
Kata:	'Watch me.' (Kata transfers a cotton ball from the tray to the jar slowly and deliberately.) 'You have a turn.' (She hands the tweezers to Ruth. Ruth takes them and after a few attempts at grasping the tweezers in different ways, picks up a cotton ball and puts it into the jar.)
Kata:	'Great, well done. Can you do another one?' (Ruth transfers another cotton ball.)

Ruth continues transferring the rest of the cotton balls with Kata's encouragement. She then agrees to take them out of the jar with the tweezers and put them back into the metal tray.

10

MUSIC

What is your favourite piece of music? Why? What emotions does the piece evoke in you?

Music is a primal and fundamental part of all human cultures, and some researchers have argued that music developed before language did. We haven't figured out why music and accompanying dance developed. Competing theories are that music evolved as a way of increasing sexual attractiveness (like the songs of songbirds), promoting group bonding (like singing a team song) or as an accidental artefact of our brains' tendency to see patterns, causing us to interpret regularly timed noises as rhythms or repeated pitches as melodies.

When we make music we usually have our attention focused in the moment even if we're drawing on information stored in our memory. Music is almost always associated with emotions, sometimes more strongly and sometimes more weakly.

I have met people with dementia who do not talk but can sing, and people with dementia who have very poor memories but who play complex pieces on the piano from memory. This is because singing a song or playing the piano uses procedural memory for music. Since procedural learning is relatively intact in people with dementia, they can also learn how to sing a new song more easily than may be expected. Choirs for people with dementia often include a mix of traditional and new songs, and the people with dementia learn to sing the new songs. Many people with dementia forget that they can make music. We once filmed a lady with dementia playing the piano. When we showed her the video later, she was surprised that it was her playing, and both proud and impressed at her own accomplishment!

If the person with dementia you care for used to play an instrument, they might still be able to do this. I would encourage you to facilitate the opportunity for them to try to play; we have seen some people become themselves again for the minutes they are playing. However, do not be disappointed if they refuse or are unable to play.

Music is a good technique for connecting with people with moderate to severe dementia who are less able to communicate verbally. Research suggests that people with dementia benefit from music more when they are actively participating, by which I mean singing, clapping or moving to the music in some other way. Getting the person with dementia physically involved makes them use their brain and their body more than if they were just passively listening.

Music is a powerful way of encouraging reminiscence. When we hear certain songs they take us back to situations when we previously heard them — a dance song reminding us of our teenage years, Christmas carols reminding us of family sing-alongs around the piano, a lullaby reminding us of our mother or our children. After participating in music, people with dementia may want to talk about the music itself, memories relating to the music or the content of the songs. Or they might be more stimulated and chatty generally.

CHOOSING MUSIC

Many of us have strong opinions about what music we like and dislike. Many people with dementia will too. Most of us like music that was popular around our formative years — age ten to 25 — though we may also enjoy a diversity of music from other styles and eras. Don't assume that a person of a certain age will like music from their era.

There are many ways of deciding what music to use with the person with dementia you care for. If you know them well, you might already know the particular pieces of music that have played a part in their life. If not, ask them or their family about what music they like. If you get vague answers, ask them more specific questions: What music was popular when you used to go to dances? What songs did you dance to with your husband? Were there any songs you used to sing as a child or that you sang to your children? What music was played at your wedding? Did you go to concerts — tell me more about those.

If you can't get specific information about the music that a person with dementia likes, then you have to go on a musical detective hunt. Try playing music they may have a connection with and watch for their reaction. Make sure that you watch for their reaction during the most catchy or memorable part of the song, such as the chorus, rather than during an instrumental introduction or verse. Once you have discovered one or two pieces that they like, you can try different pieces of the same style, or same artist or same era. You could start by trying music that was popular in their country of birth during their formative years (when they were aged between ten and 25) or songs that many people may know because of high popularity such as childhood songs, Christmas carols, hymns, traditional songs and classical music. There is a list of these pieces of music for English-speaking countries at the end of this chapter.

Case study

BRIAN

Brian is attended to but not warmly spoken of by the care staff. When they interact with him, he is either minimally responsive or irritated. He demonstrates little warmth or humour with them.

One of the care staff looking after Brian, Angie, decides to try to connect with him through music. She tries to find out what kind of music he likes but June and Gary don't know. She tries music from his youth such as Motown and Big Band but he doesn't respond much. One day she notices him tapping his foot to a country and western song that plays as the background music to a television program. So she borrows an old country and western CD from the library. She plays it for him and he taps along. He starts singing along to *The Days of Old Khancoban* by Smoky Dawson; he continues to listen and react to the rest of the music. At the end of the CD, Angie plays *The Days of Old Khancoban* for him again and once again he sings along, and she tries to hum along with him. Angie says: 'Do you like this music?' to which Brian responds, 'A great song.'

'Would you like to listen to his music again tomorrow?' asks Angie. 'Yes,' says Brian, and he gives Angie a big smile, which is unusual from him.

From then on, whenever Angie is working she plays old country music to Brian. He seems to like Smoky Dawson and Slim Dusty best, but enjoys modern country such as Keith Urban as well. The other staff remark about how

Brian seems to be more relaxed and comes out of his shell more when the music is playing. If he is in a cranky mood he might continue to pace and hum and tap along, but the music seems to calm him down. So, when Brian is uncooperative with showering or dressing, Angie sings *The Days of Old Khancoban* to him, and often he sings along and becomes more agreeable. Sometimes she encourages him to clap or tap the table in time to the music, and he often goes along with this.

Angie talks with Gary and June about Brian enjoying music, and writes down a list of music that he seems to particularly like. June puts the songs on Angie's list onto an iPod. They try several sets of headphones before they find a pair that is comfortable enough so that Brian won't pull them off. Every day staff put the music on for him, and he seems to know what it means when he sees the headphones, most times accepting them and enjoying listening to the music. This continues even when his dementia deteriorates.

The above example shows how an observant carer who spends time with a person with dementia can find out the type of music that interests them. It shows how Angie was able to interact with Brian through music and build their relationship. Systematic observation (and possibly documentation) of a person's reactions to music can help create a tailored playlist for them. It shows that when staff see a person with dementia as having an interest or hobby, it can make them seem more like a person, in the same way that finding out some personal information about a stranger can make you feel more familiar with them. It also shows the benefits of setting up a system so that all staff could give Brian access to his music. This illustrates how good communication and responsiveness between family and professional carers helps in developing and delivering activities.

Residents who are more cranky or behaviourally challenging, or who demand more time than staff can give, may receive less affection from staff. If a resident responds easily when spoken to or touched, and the carer gets some satisfaction from the response, the resident receives more attention and responds even more positively. On the other hand, if the resident does not respond easily to staff, he or she receives less attention. If staff find or are shown a way to interact with residents so that they are responsive, the resident may receive more positive attention. Staff might think that residents will only response positively with family because they have an established relationship, but if they see other staff members having positive interactions with the resident they might be more likely to try to interact with them in an engagement-focused rather than a task-focused way.

SOURCING MUSIC

If you are in luck, the person with dementia might already have an old record collection that you can rummage through, in which case you just need to locate a working turntable and you're in music. If you're looking for specific pieces of music or lyrics for songs, these may be available on iTunes, on YouTube or other sites on the internet. If you're looking for genres of music, or music from specific artists or eras, you may also be able to find these pieces through your local library. There may also be free-to-air or internet radio stations playing music of specific genres or eras.

When looking for music, if there is an 'original' version of a song that the person would have listened to a lot, preferentially use that over a cover version. The internet has made it much easier to access old music and lesser known music. Local libraries also have music collections of varying size and depth. This makes is much easier to find music that a person with dementia may relate to.

Remember that you carry a musical instrument around all the time — your voice! Some of you might think that you can't sing. You can sing, though you might not like the sound of your own singing. The point of singing to, and hopefully with, a person with dementia is not to put on an award-winning performance. Your singing will almost certainly be good enough for the person with dementia — and if they are critical of your singing then you've provoked a response, though perhaps not the intended one! Singing is a really convenient way of engaging a person with dementia when you're doing another task with them. Professional carers have told me about how when they sing with the person with dementia, they are happier and more cooperative when getting dressed or having a shower.

PRESENTING MUSIC

You can use music to stimulate, energize and activate the person with dementia, or to distract and calm them down. You can choose different music depending on what your intention is, or you might find that the same pieces work for both situations. Use the same pieces of music repeatedly; as the person becomes more and more familiar with the music they will relax into the music even more. If you're going to use a portable music player and headphones, as have been shown to be effective for nursing-home residents in providing diversion and enjoyment, make sure you use comfortable headphones fitted to the person and that the volume is at an appropriate level for their hearing.

Sing

Sing together, either *a capella* or to recorded music. If you don't know the words, hum along, look them up or make them up. It doesn't matter if you think you have a terrible voice or you think you can't hold a tune — as long as the person with dementia doesn't complain about your singing then keep doing it!

If the person with dementia can't sing the whole song, he may be able to sing the chorus or just parts of the chorus, in which case cue them into their part. For example, as part of the song *He's Got the Whole World in His Hands* he might sing 'in his hands'.

Move

When singing or just listening to music, encourage the person to move to the music. Model the movements you want them to do and get him to copy you — some of these can be done either standing or sitting, and you can do a combination of these. The person is exercising their brain when copying your behaviour, coordinating their movements and synchronizing them to the music. For example:

- clap your hands or clap your thighs, or alternate between these
- snap your fingers
- stamp or march your feet
- sway from side to side

- hold hands and swing them forward and back
- raise your arms up above your head and back down again (like flying)
- dance.

Case study

JOY

Bernie has dusted off their old record collection and taken out the turntable. After changing the needle he pulls out one of Joy's old favourites, *Ella Fitzgerald Sings the Cole Porter Song Book* and puts it on. The chorus starts for the first song: 'All through the night, I delight in your love, All through the night you're so close to me! All through the night!' Joy comes in humming and Bernie spontaneously grabs her hands and pulls her into a dance hold. They start dancing together and dance through the whole of the first side.

After the last dance, they collapse onto the lounge.

Joy: 'You're still a great dancer.'

Bernie: 'So are you.'

Joy: 'I always like dancing with you. You used to sweep us around the dance floor.'

Bernie: 'I had to be good or all the other lads would have claimed you.'

Joy: 'No ...'

Bernie: 'Yes, there were many times when I danced you away from a gentleman who looked as

	if he might like to cut in. It was those long legs of yours.'
Joy:	'My legs are still long.'
Bernie:	'Yes they are, and you are as lovely to dance with then as you are now.'
Joy:	(hugging him) 'Bernie ...'
Bernie:	'I'm so glad I've got you.'
Joy:	'I'm so glad I've got you.'

The above example shows how music led to spontaneous dancing (exercise!), reminiscence and physical and emotional closeness. Putting the music on took them out of their routine interactions and stimulated some old memories and associated romantic feelings.

POPULAR SONGS FROM THE PAST

Here is a list of artists and songs from the 1930s, 1940s and 1950s. Pick songs from the era when the person was aged between ten and 25 years. I'm aware that this is a very Western-centric list, and that people from other cultures might have different music they will have listened to during their youth.

Song	Artist	Year
Happy Days are Here Again	Ben Selvin	1930
Puttin' on the Ritz	Harry Richman	1930
Minnie the Moocher	Cab Calloway and his Cotton Club Orchestra	1931
Night and Day	Fred Astaire and Leo Reisman	1932

Song	Artist	Year
All of Me	Louis Armstrong	1932
Moonglow	Benny Goodman	1934
Smoke Gets in Your Eyes	Paul Whiteman	1934
Cheek to Cheek	Fred Astaire	1935
Pennies from Heaven	Bing Crosby	1936
The Way You Look Tonight	Fred Astaire	1936
Sing, Sing, Sing (With a Swing)	Benny Goodman	1937
One O'Clock Jump	Count Basie	1937
They Can't Take That Away From Me	Fred Astaire	1937
Begin the Beguine	Artie Shaw	1938
A-Tisket A-Tasket	Ella Fitzgerald	1938
Bei Mir Bist Du Schoen	The Andrews Sisters	1938
Over the Rainbow	Judy Garland	1939
Moonlight Serenade	Glenn Miller	1939
God Bless America	Kate Smith	1939
Strange Fruit	Billie Holiday	1939
In the Mood	Glenn Miller	1940
Chattanooga Choo Choo	Glenn Miller	1941
White Christmas	Bing Crosby	1942
Swinging on a Star	Bing Crosby	1944
Don't Fence Me In	Bing Crosby and The Andrews Sisters	1944
I'll Be Seeing You	Bing Crosby	1944
Rum and Coco-Cola	The Andrews Sisters	1945
Sentimental Journey	Les Brown and Doris Day	1945
Prisoner of Love	Perry Como	1946
Buttons and Bows	Dinah Shore	1948
I'm Looking Over a Four Leaf Clover	Art Mooney	1948
Riders in the Sky	Vaughn Monroe	1949
Rudolph the Red-nosed Reindeer	Gene Autry	1949
Theme from The Third Man	Anton Karas	1950

Song	Artist	Year
Mona Lisa	Nat King Cole	1950
(Put Another Nickel in) Music! Music! Music!	Teresa Brewer	1950
Too Young	Nat King Cole	1951
Unforgettable	Nat King Cole	1951
You Belong To Me	Jo Stafford	1952
Here in My Heart	Al Martino	1952
Auf Wiederseh'n Sweetheart	Vera Lynn	1952
Vaya Con Dios (May God Be With You)	Les Paul and Mary Ford	1953
Mister Sandman	The Chordettes	1954
Secret Love	Doris Day	1954
Rock Around the Clock	Bill Haley and his Comets	1955
Que Sera Sera (Whatever Will Be Will Be)	Doris Day	1956
Blueberry Hill	Fats Domino	1956
Hound Dog	Elvis Presley	1956
Jailhouse Rock	Elvis Presley	1957
Great Balls of Fire	Jerry Lee Lewis	1957
The Kingston Trio	Tom Dooley	1958
Mack the Knife	Bobby Darin	1959

OTHER POPULAR SONGS

Here are some other popular genres and songs you might like to try:

Nursery rhymes

- *Ring a Ring a Rosie*
- *Baa Baa Black Sheep*
- *Old McDonald Had a Farm*
- *Hickory Dickory Dock*
- *Row Row Row your Boat*
- *Twinkle Twinkle Little Star*

Christmas carols

- *Jingle Bells*
- *Silent Night*
- *We Wish You a Merry Christmas*
- *Joy to the World*
- *Away in a Manger*
- *We Three Kings*

Traditional songs

- *Waltzing Matilda*
- *When Irish Eyes are Smiling*
- *Scarborough Fair*
- *Danny Boy*
- *The Road to Gundagai*
- *Yankee Doodle*
- *She'll be Coming Round the Mountain*
- *When the Saints Come Marching In*

Hymns

- *Amazing Grace*
- *Ave Maria*
- *The Lord is my Shepherd*

CLASSICAL MUSIC

There are many, many pieces of classical music to choose from: here are just a few. I've chosen these because they have immediately familiar beginnings, are heard regularly on classical channels and on advertisements and television, and have regular rhythms and are easy to clap or hum to.

- Strauss, *The Blue Danube*
- Beethoven, *Symphony No. 5*
- Tchaikovsky, *Dance of the Sugar Plum Fairy*
- Beethoven, *Für Elise*
- Pachelbel's *Canon.*

11

PLAY

When was the last time you played?

Adult responsibilities such as earning a living, maintaining a household and caring for others seem much more important than playing. Caring for a person in particular takes so much energy and time that it may seem impossible to consider wasting time playing. As we get older most of us play less and less. We prioritize work over play. However, as Brian Sutton-Smith of Harvard University writes: 'The opposite of play is not work, it is depression.'

Play isn't any specific activity — it is a state of activity. We can play at work, and for some, work is play.

PLAY IS GOOD FOR US

Play has been shown to be critical to the development of children. Here are some of the benefits of play in children:

- contributes to healthy brain development
- allows them to explore the world
- gives them opportunities to practise roles (e.g. leader, teacher, doctor)

- encourages them to develop new skills, build confidence and resilience
- fosters creativity, flexibility and learning
- builds social skills and connections
- encourages physical activity and physical development
- lets them practise decision-making skills
- helps them discover their own interests and sense of self.

There is increasing evidence that play is also important for adults. Play strengthens bonds and enhances relationships, improves creativity and productivity, and improves mental health. People who are more playful are also rated as more attractive. The benefits of play for adults has been recognized and acted upon by some innovative organizations such as Google, YouTube and Twitter. All these organizations encourage their employees to play at work because this improves mood and fosters productivity and creativity. More extreme examples of organizations' attempts to facilitate play at work include the provision of scooters, ping pong tables, a photo booth, giant slides and a 'barefoot in the office' policy. More common examples of fostering play at work are casual dress days, team-building exercises, organized lunchtime sport or after-work drinks. These activities seem to suggest that play is an activity; however, the intent is that the activity stimulates a state of play and the playfulness continues into work activities.

Adult recreational play is often described as doing specific activities such as participating in a sports, music or book club, going to a party or event, playing an instrument, or learning some new skill like a language or craft. However, when we think about what play is we realize that it doesn't have to occur only in relation to specific activities. Children play constantly and can make any activity a game or play.

Stewart Brown, founder of the National Institute for Play in the United States, says that play is:

- apparently purposeless (done for its own sake)
- voluntary
- inherently attractive — fun, interesting, you want to do it
- free from time — you lose sense of time when playing
- free from sense of self — you stop being self-conscious when you're playing, and you can be someone else when playing
- something that provides opportunities to improvise, be spontaneous, try things in different ways
- something you want to keep doing.

What the science tells us

Work on humour therapy with people with dementia shows us that they still play. Our research group at the University of New South Wales conducted the Sydney Multisite Intervention of LaughterBosses and ElderClowns (SMILE) study, which involved trained performers visiting residents in nursing homes, assisted by trained staff members. Our research showed that humour therapy decreased agitation in people with dementia living in nursing homes. We also found that the more the person enjoyed the humour visits and the more sessions they received, the more their levels of agitation and depression decreased and their quality of life improved.

Other researchers have shown that people with moderate dementia enjoy and can successfully create and perform stand-up comedy.

Case study

RUTH

Ruth's daughter Julie thought during a visit to Ruth she would do a fashion-related activity and have some fun with her mother.

Julie:	'Mum, I need some advice. I'm going to the races this weekend and I need to choose a hat and some accessories.' (Julie takes a cowboy hat out of the bag and puts it on her head.)
Julie:	'What do you think about this one?'
Ruth:	'No, that's a boy's one.'
Julie:	(puts on a beret and pulls a snooty face) 'Parlez-vous français?'
Ruth:	(smiles) 'That's a French hat.'
Julie:	'I think it looks nice on me.'
Ruth:	'Yes.' (Julie puts the beret on Ruth's head and takes out a hand mirror.)
Julie:	'It looks nice on you too, Mum.' (Ruth looks at herself in the mirror, tilts her head and smiles. Julie puts a dirty baseball cap on her own head, crosses her arms and leans back and makes a tough face.)
Julie:	'Do you like this one on me, Mum?'
Ruth:	'No.' (Julie puts on a straw sunhat with pink roses, rests her chin on her palms.)
Julie:	'How about this one?'

Ruth:	'That's better.'
Julie:	'I think this would look good on you.' (puts the straw hat on Ruth's head.)
Ruth:	(smiles at herself in the mirror) 'Yes, that's for me.'
Julie:	'You look like a duchess.' (curtseys) 'Hello m'lady.'
Ruth:	(smiles and holds out her hand regally) 'Hello ...'

The interaction continues with several more hats, then with some necklaces.

The above example shows how people with dementia can and will play. The point of the exercise was to interact and have fun. Julie's approach was critical in that she was dramatically playful from the start, with her snooty face and French words. Ruth understood that it was play-acting and played along. The hats gave Ruth an additional cue to following Julie's play-acting.

PLAYING WITH PEOPLE WITH DEMENTIA

Play is such a fundamental part of human behaviour, it should be no surprise that people with dementia can still play and are often very open to playing. Similar to when doing creative activities, people with dementia often surprise us in their ability to play. They just need the opportunities and encouragement to do so. Playing regularly with people with dementia seems to improve their behaviour and may improve their mood.

When you invite a person with dementia to play with you, you're implicitly valuing them as a person who is good company. You can plan playful activities for people with dementia, and you can also look out for spontaneous opportunities to play with them. Being playful means being in the moment, and looking for opportunities to play means that we have to temporarily put aside worries or stresses of the moment, or temporarily delay other tasks we need to complete. Some of you may naturally and easily find this 'playful' attitude. If you're not one of these lucky few, no matter, you can work on it. These playful moments may be short, just one or two minutes. As with everything, as you practise being more playful it becomes easier and will start to be second nature.

Pitch the play to the cognitive abilities of the person with dementia. A person with better cognition may appreciate a joke or pun. A person with very poor cognition might find a funny face or peekaboo game amusing. Here are some ideas to get you started playing with a person with dementia:

- Tell a story or a joke related to the situation
  e.g. 'This queue is so long we could have grown a beard by the time we get to the front' or 'You've been married 50 years? I don't believe it, you must have been five when you got married!' or 'I remember the time I was in a queue in South America ...' (story continues).
- Play a simple or familiar game like asking which cup the bean is under, or flipping a coin for heads or tails.
- Make an ordinary activity into a game — you could play the game while the person watches or they can play along with you (e.g. avoid the cracks in the pavement while walking, look for red flowers while out for a walk, or race while podding the peas or folding the clothes).

- Try to make the person laugh by doing something in a silly, funny or exaggerated way, e.g. walking in a funny way, putting a bowl on your head and pulling a funny face, or popping your head around the corner (like when playing peekaboo) and 'disappearing' quickly when they see you.
- Set up play between two people, encouraging the person with dementia to watch. For instance, tell the person with dementia that you are 'hiding' from another person because you're in trouble, then hide. The other person (who is in on the game) comes to find you and makes exaggerated comments about what trouble you will be in when they find you. See whether or not the person with dementia reveals where you are hiding. Or start a silly argument between two people (e.g. whether cats or dogs are better) and ask the person with dementia to judge who wins the debate.

In order to play with people with dementia you might need to relearn how to be playful. I believe that we fall out of practice playing, and by playing more we can get in practice again. I wish that being silly didn't have negative connotations. Adults are often reluctant to play because they don't want to seem silly. We need to stop worrying about looking silly when we play; being silly for a while doesn't mean you're a silly person or less worthwhile in other ways.

Here are some things to do to get your playfulness going.

- Play with children, they are experts on play.
- Watch a funny movie or read a funny book.
- Play a board game or other type of game, preferably with other people.
- Plan a surprise for someone.

- Make something: music, art, a cake, a garden box, a mess!
- Do something you've wanted to but haven't because it's silly — jump in puddles, eat a lollypop, lick your plate, get dressed up and dance around the house.
- Do something spontaneous that is fun.
- Remember times when you have been cheeky or mischievous and try to capture that feeling again.

PLAY AND HUMOUR SHOULD NOT BE HURTFUL

Sometimes play or humour can go too far. For instance, a physical game could get rough so that one of the participants gets hurt. Similarly, play and humour can be hurtful rather than pleasurable and funny. It is important when playing to be aware of boundaries of safe play. Try to avoid play where someone is the victim, such as someone being the butt of a joke. For instance, avoid making jokes or teasing the person with dementia about their memory or cognitive abilities. Avoid play that is nasty, mean-spirited, hostile or aggressive.

Case study

ANTONIO

Maria has realized that Antonio doesn't smile much anymore. He smiles in the face, but not from within. She decides to try to tease and laugh with him more often.

Maria: 'Antonio?'

Antonio: 'Yes, *cucciola mia*?'

Maria: 'You look very handsome today.' (smiles slyly at him)

Antonio: 'I do?'

Maria: 'Yes, as handsome as when we first met. Maybe even more handsome.'

Antonio: 'No, no, I am old now.'

Maria: 'Only in age, not in body ... Stand up and let me see you.' (Antonio stands up)

Maria: 'Turn around.' (Antonio turns around a little hesitantly)

Maria: 'Hmm ...' (looking him up and down, takes him by the hand)

Maria: 'You are right, you look older. You were 40 when we met, you look at least 43 now.'

Antonio: '43 ...'

Maria: Actually, 43 and a half ...'

Antonio: 'That half is important for my maturity ...' (smiles)

Maria: 'Handsome and mature. *Perfetto.*'

Antonio: 'You are *perfetto.* You look after me so well.' (squeezes her hand)

Maria: 'Will you dance with me, handsome? We haven't danced for ages. Wait, I will put on the music.'

Antonio and Maria dance together.

This example shows a playful, humorous and affectionate interaction. Initiated and led by Maria, Antonio also makes a joke as part of the conversation. The interaction reminds both Maria and Antonio of their early romance and also their long shared history.

A FEW LAST WORDS

I hope this book has given you ideas and inspiration as well as some practical tips on developing and delivering engaging activities for people with dementia. Remember that in order to flourish psychologically, both you and the person you care for need to experience three positive emotions to every one negative emotion, so create opportunities to have positive experiences. I hope that in applying these ideas there will be more smiles in your days.

FURTHER RESOURCES

Here are the contact details for some further resources you might find helpful.

National associations

Dementia Australia
www.dementia.org.au

Alzheimer Society Canada
http://www.alzheimer.ca/en

Alzheimers New Zealand
www.alzheimers.org.nz

Alzheimer's Society UK
www.alzheimers.org.uk

Alzheimer's Association USA
www.alz.org

Other resources

Artists for Alzheimer's (ARTZ)
This US organization links art to people with dementia and their carers. They developed the art gallery and museum partnership program and also have circus, film and poetry projects for people with dementia: www.artistsforalzheimers.org

ARTZ UK
www.progamsforelderly.com/memory-artz-artists-for-alhemiers-uk.php

Arts 4 Dementia
A UK organization that creates opportunities for people with dementia and their carers to experience the arts including dance, music and poetry: www.arts4dementia.org.uk

Dementia Australia (Montessori activities)

Go to www.dementia.org.au and type 'Montessori activities' in the search box.

Arts Health Institute

An Australian organization that provides arts programs in health care, including a humour program for nursing homes: www.artshealthinstitute.org.au

Australian Men's Shed Association

This website also has links to Men's Shed websites in other countries: www.mensshed.org

Centre for Applied Research in Dementia

Information from Cameron Camp, the originator of Montessori activities for people with dementia, including the purchase of manuals and books: www.cen4ard.com/index.php

Cognitive Stimulation Therapy

Information on cognitive stimulation therapy, including how to buy the manuals: www.cstdementia.com

Creative Dementia Arts Network

A UK knowledge and practice hub for those involved in arts and dementia: www.creativedementia.org

Generations United Tried and True guide

A guide for creating successful intergenerational activities for nursing-home residents and preschool children: www.intergenerational.clahs.vt.edu/pdf/jarrotttriedtrue.pdf

Life history books

Information on how to create a life history book, and a life history book template: www.alzheimers.org.uk/site/scripts/download_info. php?fileID=1434

Go to www.dementia.org.au and type 'life history book' in the search box.

Music & Memory

A US organization that provides personalized music to older people using iPods, and provides training for family and professional carers:

www.musicandmemory.org/about/mission-and-vision

Society for the Arts in Dementia Care

A Canadian organization that promotes creative expression in dementia care: www.cecd-society.org

Talking Mats

A tool to facilitate communication with people who have communication difficulties: www.talkingmats.com

TimeSlips

Information on a creative storytelling program:
www.timeslips.org/about

Tourism For All

A UK organization offering accessible services and facilities to everyone; their website has a page listing organizations that offer services for people with dementia:

www.tourismforall.org.uk/Alzheimers-and-dementia-holidays. html

Toilet maps

When planning outings the following toilet maps might be useful. Local tourist information offices might also be able to help you find toilets if you're visiting an area you are unfamiliar with.

Australia: www.toiletmap.gov.au

Britain: www.greatbritishpublictoiletmap.rca.ac.uk

New Zealand: www.toiletmap.co.nz

New York: www.nyrestroom.com

BIBLIOGRAPHY

Ahlskog, J.E., Geda, Y.E., et al., 2011, 'Physical Exercise as a Preventive or Disease-Modifying Treatment of Dementia and Brain Aging', Mayo Clinic Proceedings 86 (9), pp. 876–884.

Algase, D.L., Beck, C., Kolanowski, A., Whall, A., Berent, S., Richards, K., and Beattie, E., 1996, 'Need-Driven Dementia-Compromised Behavior: An Alternative View of Disruptive Behavior', *American Journal of Alzheimer's Disease and Other Dementias*, vol. 11 (6), pp. 10–19.

Brodaty, H. and Arasaratnam, C., 2012, 'Meta-Analysis of Nonpharmacological Interventions for Neuropsychiatric Symptoms of Dementia', *American Journal of Psychiatry*, vol. 169 (9), pp. 946–53.

Buettner, L. and Kolanowski, A., 2003, 'Practice Guidelines for Recreation Therapy in the Care of People with Dementia', *Geriatric Nursing*, vol. 24 (1), pp. 18–25.

Cohen-Mansfield, J., Dakheel-Ali, M. and Marx, M.S., 2009, 'Engagement in Persons with Dementia: The Concept and Its Measurement', *American Journal of Geriatric Psychiatry*, vol. 17 (4), pp. 299–307.

Cohen-Mansfield, J., Thein, K., Dakheel-Ali, M. and Marx, M.S., 2010, 'The Underlying Meaning of Stimuli: Impact on Engagement of Persons with Dementia', *Psychiatry Research*, vol. 177 (1–2), pp. 216–22.

Cohen-Mansfield, J., Thein, K., Marx, M.S., Dakheel-Ali, M. and Freedman, L., 2012, 'Efficacy of Nonpharmacologic Interventions for Agitation in Advanced Dementia: A Randomized, Placebo-Controlled Trial', *Journal of Clinical Psychiatry*, vol. 73 (9), pp. 1255–61.

Egan, M.Y., Munroe, S., Hubert, C., Rossiter, T., Gauthier, A., Eisner, M., Fulford, N., Neilson, M., Daros, B. and Rodrigue,

C., 2007, 'Caring for Residents with Dementia and Aggressive Behavior: Impact of Life History Knowledge', *Journal of Gerontological Nursing*, vol. 33 (2), pp. 24–30.

Epstein, A.S. and Boisvert, C., 2006, 'Let's Do Something Together: Identifying the Effective Components of Intergenerational Programs', *Journal of Intergenerational Relationships*, vol. 4 (3), pp. 87–109.

Gitlin, L.N., Winter, L., Burke, J., Chernett, N., Dennis, M.P. and Hauck, W.W., 2008, 'Tailored Activities to Manage Neuropsychiatric Behaviors in Persons with Dementia and Reduce Caregiver Burden: A Randomized Pilot Study', *American Journal of Geriatric Psychiatry*, vol. 16 (3), pp. 229–39.

Gronstedt, H., Frandin, K., Bergland, A., Helbostad, J.L., Granbo, R., Puggaard, L., Andresen, M. and Hellstrom, K., 2013, 'Effects of Individually Tailored Physical and Daily Activities in Nursing Home Residents on Activities of Daily Living, Physical Performance and Physical Activity Level: A Randomized Controlled Trial', *Gerontology*, vol. 59 (3), pp. 220–29.

Judge, K.S., Camp, C.J. and Orsulic-Jeras, S., 2000, 'Use of Montessori-Based Activities for Clients with Dementia in Adult Day Care: Effects on Engagement', *American Journal of Alzheimer's Disease*, vol. 15 (1), pp. 42–6.

Kolanowski, A., Buettner, L., Litaker, M. and Yu, F., 2006, 'Factors That Relate to Activity Engagement in Nursing Home Residents', *American Journal of Alzheimer's Disease and Other Dementias*, vol. 21 (1), pp. 15–22.

Low, L.F., Brodaty, H., Goodenough, B., Spitzer, P., Bell, J.P., Fleming, R., Casey, A.N., Liu, Z. and Chenoweth, L., 2013, 'The Sydney Multisite Intervention of Laughterbosses and

Elderclowns (Smile) Study: Cluster Randomised Trial of Humour Therapy in Nursing Homes', *BMJ Open*, vol. 3 (1).

O'Connor, D.W., Ames, D., Gardner, B. and King, M., 2009, 'Psychosocial Treatments of Behavior Symptoms in Dementia: A Systematic Review of Reports Meeting Quality Standards', *International Psychogeriatrics*, vol. 21 (02), pp. 225–40.

O'Connor, D.W., Ames, D., Gardner, B. and King, M., 2009, 'Psychosocial Treatments of Psychological Symptoms in Dementia: A Systematic Review of Reports Meeting Quality Standards', *International Psychogeriatrics*, vol. 21 (02), pp. 241–51.

Pinquart, M. and Forstmeier, S., 2012, 'Effects of Reminiscence Interventions on Psychosocial Outcomes: A Meta-Analysis', *Aging and Mental Health*, vol. 16 (5), pp. 541–58.

Raglio, A., Bellelli, G., Mazzola, P., Bellandi, D., Giovagnoli, A.R., Farina, E., Stramba-Badiale, M., Gentile, S., Gianelli, M.V., Ubezio, M.C., Zanetti, O. and Trabucchi, M., 2012, 'Music, Music Therapy and Dementia: A Review of Literature and the Recommendations of the Italian Psychogeriatric Association', *Maturitas*, vol. 72 (4), pp. 305–10.

Ritchie, K. and Lovestone, S., 2002, 'The Dementias', *Lancet*, vol. 360 (9347), pp. 1767–69.

Ward, R., Howorth, M., Wilkinson, H., Campbell, S. and Keady, J., 2012, 'Supporting the Friendships of People with Dementia', *Dementia*, vol. 11 (3), pp. 287–303.

Woods, B., Aguirre, E., Spector, A.E. and Orrell, M., 2012, 'Cognitive Stimulation to Improve Cognitive Functioning in People with Dementia', *Cochrane Database of Systematic Reviews (Online)*, vol. 2.

INDEX

physical health, area of unmet need 26-7
piano playing 205-6
places of significance
    Antonio's story 44, 60
    Brian's story 52
    Joy's story 40, 58
    life history component 36
    Ruth's story 48
planning
    difficulties with 18-20
    writing down steps 20
play
    benefits of 218-20
    possible options 222
    should not be hurtful 225
    what it is 219-20
    at work 219
pleasure, experiencing 4-6
praise, regular 100
problem solving, difficulties with 18-20
procedural memory 123, 205-6
prospective memory 12-3
psychological symptoms 26-7
public acceptance 186-7
public toilets map 233
puzzles 115-6

R
reflecting back, in conversations 135
relationships, changing nature of 6-8
reminiscence
    control of conversation 134
    life review 126-9
    moderate–severe dementia 141-9
    risks to 129
    simple 128, 130-3
residential care see nursing homes
restaurants, dementia-specific 180
restroom map 233
routines
    mentally stimulating 121-5
    pros and cons 109

Ruth's story
    activity calendar 108
    current thinking abilities 50-1
    increased visits 159-64
    knitting activity 75-8
    life history components 48-9
    nursing-related activities 202-4
    plays with hats 221-2
    potential activities 61-3

S
secrets, revealing 129
self-care, systematic modification 195-6
self-censor, lose ability to 23-4
self-identity, maintaining 9
self-reflection 102
sensory stimulation 114
serotonin, increasing levels 5
setting the table 196
short-term memory
    assessment table 32
    limited size 11
    memory aids 13-4
sight, assessing 33
singing 205-6, 211-2
skill, areas for improvement 103-4
smell, impaired ability 22
soccer, grandson talking about 172-3
social isolation 151-2
social network
    concentric circles 152
    losing 151-2
social status, changes in 93-5
socialising, with friends 159
Society for the Arts in Dementia Care 233
solutions, difficulty creating 19
songs, list of popular songs 214-7
sorting category related games 116
spaced retrieval technique 124
speech, difficulties with 21
stigma, dealing with 186-7
stimulation
    area of unmet need 26-7